Childhood Obesity

CURRENT CONCEPTS IN NUTRITION

Myron Winick, Editor

Institute of Human Nutrition
Columbia University College of Physicians and Surgeons

Volume 1: Nutrition and Development

Volume 2: Nutrition and Fetal Development

Volume 3: Childhood Obesity

CHILDHOOD OBESITY

Edited by

MYRON WINICK

Institute of Human Nutrition
Columbia University College of Physicians and Surgeons

A WILEY-INTERSCIENCE PUBLICATION

JOHN WILEY & SONS
New York • London • Sydney • Toronto

Copyright © 1975 by John Wiley & Sons, Inc.

All rights reserved. Published simultaneously in Canada.

No part of this book may be reproduced by any means, nor transmitted, nor translated into a machine language without the written permission of the publisher.

Library of Congress Cataloging in Publication Data:

Winick, Myron.
 Childhood obesity.

 (Current concepts in nutrition ; v. 3)
 "A Wiley-Interscience publication."
 Includes index.
 1. Corpulence in children. I. Title. II. Series.

RJ399.C6W55   618.9′23′98   75-1173
ISBN 0-471-95441-1

Printed in the United States of America

10 9 8 7 6 5 4 3 2 1

Preface

Obesity, one of the main health problems in America today, also constitutes a significant health hazard in developing countries. It is not, therefore, a disease of affluence alone, of simple overeating, but a widely prevalent form of malnutrition. The more we learn about obesity, the more it becomes obvious that, as is true of other types of malnutrition, there are periods in life when an individual is particularly vulnerable. One such period is childhood. Not only is the child at risk, but the kind of obesity he develops may be particularly dangerous for it may sentence him to a lifetime of obesity.

Research is beginning to suggest that at least one type of adult obesity may be induced in early life. An interaction of genetic factors and early nutritional experience may program the number of fat cells within the various fat depots. Once this program has been written it may be extremely difficult if not impossible to rewrite it.

This volume reviews the evidence leading to this conclusion. It probes such questions as the cellular differences between early-onset and later-onset obesity and discusses the prevalence of early-onset obesity, its causes, and the methods currently being used for prevention and therapy. No real answers are available and therefore much of the material is controversial. But at present knowledge in this area is proliferating very rapidly and the authors of the various chapters are in the forefront of gathering that new knowledge.

Any volume dealing with a problem as complex as this one must of course be selective. Not all areas of childhood obesity are covered. What has been attempted is to choose those areas that are rapidly progressing, to relate them to other areas of research, to examine their relevance to clinically important matters, and to put into perspective at this moment in time the importance of childhood obesity as a world health problem.

MYRON WINICK, M.D.

New York, New York
February 1975

08258

v

Contents

Childhood Obesity

Introduction

MYRON WINICK, M.D.

Institute of Human Nutrition, College of Physicians and Surgeons,
Columbia University, New York, New York

The conference on childhood obesity was the second annual symposium on nutrition held by the Institute of Human Nutrition of Columbia University, College of Physicians and Surgeons. Its purpose was to bring together a group of physicians and biochemists to discuss what we are beginning to believe may be a very dangerous form of obesity, childhood obesity.

The conference began with a discussion of certain cellular and tissue changes that may be unique to "early-onset" obesity, progressed to observations on the clinical picture of obesity in infants, children, and adolescents, and a discussion of some of the major long-term consequences of obesity in early life. The conference closed with a discussion of treatment from the standpoint of dietary management, hormones, and behavioral modification.

Jules Hirsch, professor of human behavior and metabolism at Rockefeller University, discussed his work on the newest concept of obesity, namely the relation of the condition to the number and size of adipose cells in both experimental and clinical obesity.

According to this point of view, the fat in the adipose tissue may be packaged in a large number of small cells or in a smaller number of larger cells. Dr. Hirsch has pioneered methods to determine cell number and cell size in adipose tissue.

The problems in methodology that still exist are related primarily to determination of total body fat, the representativeness of any one biopsy site, and the fact that an "adipocyte" can be recognized only after fat has

1

begun to accumulate. Nevertheless, classification according to relative number and size of fat cells is regarded by many as a major breakthrough in our understanding of the fundamental tissue changes that take place in obesity. Early in his studies, Dr. Hirsch noted that the adipocytes of nonobese individuals averaged 0.6 to 0.7 mg of fat per cell, whereas those of obese individuals averaged about 20% more. Further, the nonobese individual had approximately three hundred billion fat cells, and the obese individual usually had about twice that number. Thus in very obese adults the really mammoth cellular difference was in the number of fat cells. When such adults lost weight, the effect at the cell level was almost entirely on cell size. Cell number changed very little, if at all.

Further studies conducted on a larger number of subjects suggested that there are two types of obesity: one wherein the patient has too many fat cells and would be said to be suffering from "hyperplastic obesity," and the other wherein the patient has fat cells that are too large, a condition called "hypertrophic obesity." It appears that early-onset (childhood) obesity is primarily hyperplastic, whereas late-onset (adult) obesity is hypertrophic. Although these findings appear to be statistically valid, there is always "overlap" in both directions; some adult-onset obesity was hyperplastic and some early-onset was hypertrophic, according to the report given by Dr. Hirsch.

To characterize these types of obesity more clearly, animal studies were undertaken. During normal growth, the number of epididymal fat-pad cells of a rat reached a maximum at around 12 weeks of age, according to the Rockefeller investigator. Nothing done to the animal after this time changed cell number. From then on, the growth of the fat was hypertrophic. He also reported that when a lesion was made in the ventromedial portion of the hypothalamus at 7 weeks of age, marked hyperphagia and obesity ensued but, again, cell number was not affected. Cell size, however, increased enormously. Thus even though new fat cells were still appearing at that time, cell number reached the same plateau as in the nonlesioned animals.

On the other hand, dietary manipulation during the first three weeks of life alters the number of fat cells. Recent experiments by Marci Greenwood (a postdoctoral fellow at the Institute of Human Nutrition, Columbia University, College of Physicians and Surgeons) have shown that cell division, as measured by thymidine incorporation into DNA, in cells destined to become adipocytes stops at about 2 to 3 weeks of age. Thus even though cell number increases by the histometric osmium method beyond 7 weeks of age, the division of fat cells actually stops long before this. These data raise important questions about human obesity because the methods currently employed to discover when the number of fat cells is determined are histometric.

Cell division may cease much earlier than we have thought. The realization that adipocytes stop dividing early in life has led to an examination of cellularity in genetic obesity. The cells of most genetically obese animals are too large, and obesity begins in the adult life of these animals. By contrast, the "Zucker" rat (named after its discoverers Lois M. Zucker and Theodore F. Zucker), a genetically obese strain with too many fat cells, becomes obese early in life. Also, manipulation of these rats' diet early in life alters the expression of their genetic obesity. Subsequent ad libitum feeding allows the gene to be expressed, but prevents the animals from being as obese as they would have been had their diet not been restricted early in life. Even genetic types of obesity, therefore, may be amenable to nutritional manipulations at critical periods of development. What are the critical periods in man? These are not yet known but, in Dr. Hirsch's opinion, the last trimester of pregnancy, the first 3 years of life, and adolescence are crucial in determining whether a person will be obese.

Stanley Garn from the Center for Human Growth and Development at the University of Michigan, Ann Arbor, examined childhood obesity in epidemiologic terms. He defined an obese person as one who is above the eighty-fifth percentile for triceps fat fold for age and sex, and a lean person as one below the fifteenth percentile in the same measurement.

Dr. Garn called attention to several physical changes characteristic of the obese child that are not usually appreciated by physicians. He said, for example, that obese boys and girls are taller than their lean peers. In addition, skeletal development is advanced in the obese youngster, giving him a body of greater skeletal mass than his peers. Whether the increase in skeletal frame results from the stimulus of having to carry more weight or whether it is a concomitant phenomenon of obesity is not known. Also, obese children show higher-than-normal levels of hemoglobin and certain vitamins in their blood. Surprisingly, they have an increase not only in fat tissue but in fat-free weight (FFW).

Obesity is influenced by socioeconomic status. The children of the poor are leaner than those of more affluent parents, and this difference is not due entirely to differences in food intake. Differences also occur in various populations. Black infants are, as a rule, fatter than white infants, but the reverse is the case in later childhood. This is true even when income levels are kept constant. Puerto Ricans are fatter than either blacks or whites at the same economic level.

Dr. Garn next spoke about the relationship between childhood and adult obesity. He pointed out that in males poverty results in thin children who become thin adults. By contrast, in females poverty appears to lead to thin children who become fat women, whereas affluence results in heavy children who become slim women. From these data, Dr. Garn attacked the theory that obesity in childhood leads to obesity in the adult. Going one step further, he took the position that since there seems to be little relation between childhood and adult obesity, the entire theory of hyperplastic and hypertrophic obesity espoused by Dr. Hirsch was open to serious question.

It must be noted that the data Dr. Garn presented were cross-sectional. The lean children studied were not the same individuals grown to obese adults. We do not know whether these adults were lean 20, 30, 40, or 50 years ago. Only longitudinal data, which are not available, can answer this question. Moreover, Dr. Garn pointed out that the poor, adult female who is obese has a low FFW. This finding is in contrast to the poor female children who have high FFW. Based on body composition, obesity in poor, adult females would appear to be of a different type than that which occurs in childhood. Could obese women have hypertrophic obesity, whereas obese children have hyperplastic obesity?

Dr. Garn elegantly described the characteristics of childhood obesity, as demonstrated by his extensive cross-sectional studies. The criteria he set forth for the obese child are extremely useful, from both a research and a clinical standpoint. In using his cross-sectional data to argue that not all fat children become fat adults, he is on good ground. But when he argues that this raises serious problems with the theory of hyperplastic and hypertrophic obesity, as enunciated by both Dr. Hirsch and Dr. Jerome Knittle of Mount Sinai Medical School in this symposium, his ground is much less firm. In fact, what suggestion there is from Dr. Garn's data is perfectly consistent with the Hirsch–Knittle hypothesis.

Although Dr. Garn was concerned with the total amount of fat and its percentage when compared to other tissues, and Dr. Hirsch was concerned with the manner in which this fat is packaged, Dr. Sami Hashim, associate professor of medicine and director of the metabolic unit of the Institute of Human Nutrition concerned himself with the quality of the fat being deposited in the obese person. He noted that although unsaturated fat will cross the placenta, little of it gets into the fetal adipose tissue, and the newborn infant has almost 100% saturated fat in his adipose depot. Within 3 months of birth, however, the infant's fat tissue will change, reflecting the fat in the diet. Since most dietary fat is made up of long, even-chained fatty acids, these are what is found in the fat cells of most people. These long-chain fatty acids are transported via the thoracic duct to the systemic circulation and then deposited in the fat.

Medium-chain triglycerides (MCT), on the other hand, are transported from the intestine, through the portal circulation, to the liver, where they are metabolized and therefore do not reach fat depots. Thus, Dr. Hashim hypothesizes, feeding MCT might be one way to treat obesity and, perhaps even more important, it would modify the rate of adipocyte cell division in childhood. The composition of the fat can be altered not only by feeding naturally occurring polyunsaturates, but by feeding synthetically made, odd-chained fatty acids. The resulting adipose cells will then contain odd-chained fatty acids in their fat globules, and will release them when necessary, for example, during starvation. In contrast to the even-numbered carbon molecules, odd-chained fatty acids can be partly broken down to glucose, sparing both glycogen and body protein. This could have important effects, especially during the growing period when preservation of body protein is essential. Dr. Hashim's work, while not yet at the "practical stages," is a new and exciting approach to the problem of childhood obesity.

We then turned our attention from fat tissue to fat people: infants, children, and adolescents. William B. Weil, Jr., professor and chairman of the Department of Human Development at Michigan State University, led off with comments on the general problems of obesity in infancy. Defining obesity in terms of weight for length and of weight gain, Dr. Weil noted that although very fat infants do not appear to die in greater numbers than their counterparts of normal weight, obese infants are more prone to respiratory infections and other illnesses. However, like so many others who have studied the subject, he felt the most important problem to be that fat infants might become fat children who, in turn, would become fat adults. He was not persuaded by Dr. Garn's data that this was not so, pointing out its cross-sectional nature. He also noted that class mobility might play a role. By this he meant that a slim girl from poor circumstances who remained slim might have been able to move upward, and would, therefore, appear in the affluent adult group. By contrast, an obese girl might have moved downward and would appear in the less advantaged adult group.

Dr. Weil then turned from this topic and called attention to some of the factors involved in the etiology of infant obesity. These include maternal weight gain during pregnancy, brain damage, overzealous bottle feeding, early introduction of certain high-caloric solid foods, and such less tangible factors as the mother's and the family physician's attitude toward weight gain. Finally, the Michigan physician cautioned that when an infant begins to gain weight too rapidly dietary therapy to prevent obesity should be instituted.

Jean Mayer, professor of nutrition at the Harvard School of Public

Health, moved the discussion to obesity in childhood. He noted that certain body types are associated with obesity and that since these body types are, he believes, inherited, there is a genetic component to obesity that must be considered. For example, he asserted, if neither parent is obese, there is only a 7% chance of the child's being obese. If one parent is obese, the chance is 40%, whereas if both parents are obese, the chances jump to 80%.

Environmental factors are also important, but as society de-emphasizes physical activity, the genetic potential has more and more chance of being expressed. According to Mayer, physical activity is by far the most important environmental variable affecting obesity. Obese children and adults often eat the same amount, he said, and usually the same nutrient proportions as their lean counterparts, but they exercise much less. Studies accompanied by motion pictures were said to show that fat girls exercised one-third less than lean girls. Other studies have shown that there is no correlation between weight gain in babies and the amount of food ingested. However, fat babies were placid and thin babies active.

Having made these observations, Dr. Mayer then discussed some of the consequences of being a fat child. He noted that such children are rejected, citing as evidence a study demonstrating that fat girls have only one-third the chance of being accepted into college that lean girls have. These societal pressures are reflected in the child's personality. Psychological testing reveals a profile similar to other types of children who have experienced prejudice and discrimination. Therapy in childhood obesity must be instituted in a number of directions simultaneously. Not only must the diet be controlled, but exercise must be increased and the child must be supported psychologically. This regimen of increased activity must be a long-term one or the obesity will recur.

Felix P. Heald, professor of pediatrics at the University of Maryland School of Medicine, reported on his studies of the obese adolescent. The hallmark of adolescence is rapid change, he said. A boy's height increases about 20%; his body mass almost doubles during this period. There is also a normal deposition of fat, especially in adolescent girls. Two historical patterns may be noted in obesity, which begins when the young girl enters adolescence. The first is a distinct family history of obesity that begins in infancy. The second is no family history of obesity, but the child commences to grow fat at about the time of some specific stressful event in her life. There are three peak periods for the development of obesity in children: late infancy, early childhood around age 6, and adolescence. As Dr. Mayer had noted, Dr. Heald agreed that literature on the subject suggests that obese children do not appear to eat more than lean children. However, he pointed out that the dietary intake data upon which the Mayer statement was based were developed from 3 to 4-hour recall interviews and are of questionable reliability, because obese children and adolescents minimize food intake as a defense mechanism. Moreover, in a study in which young patients were hospitalized and fed what they indicated was their normal intake, they lost weight. These data, however, are in contrast to the one observational study done on teenagers. That study indicated that the obese eat no more than the lean. It would seem, then, that even the most basic question about childhood obesity—Does the obese child eat more than the lean child?—is not yet answered. One interesting observation on obese teenagers, however, is that they do not eat when they are hungry, but rather when they are bored. Examination of obese adolescents reveals that, although they are taller than their peers and their skeletal age is somewhat beyond their body age, they grow up to be less tall adults. Puberty comes earlier. We do not know what psychological effect this 1-year shortening of childhood has on these children. Obese children are rarely hypertensive but errors of measurement may occur if the arms are very fat.

Since adolescence is an anabolic period and weight reduction is a catabolic process, the teenager is particularly sensitive to weight reduction, Heald continued. Thus weight loss must occur very slowly, in order to preserve growth. This makes treatment of the obese adolescent particularly difficult. Not only must weight reduction be gradual, but therapy is difficult because of the poor body image of most persons whose obesity began in adolescence. That is to say, one's perception of one's own body as unattractive is shown to have begun during adolescence. This poor body image is associated with other behavioral problems that can complicate therapy. Although some improvement can be made during adolescence, Dr. Heald thinks that therapy should be aimed at prevention. It is evident that one of the major concerns with childhood obesity is the fact that these juvenile-onset obese individuals are destined to have the most severe and the most difficult to treat type of obesity when they grow up.

Another concern was the relation between the fat content of the child's diet and the hyperlipidemias so commonly seen in our adult populations.

A. K. Khachadurian, professor of medicine at Rutgers Medical School, discussed the diagnosis and management of hyperlipidemia in children. After describing the current classification of hyperlipidemias, he focused his attention on the type of primary or genetic hyperlipidemia most commonly found in the pediatric age group, namely, familial hypercholesterolemia. Homozygotes with this disease show plasma cholesterol values approximately four times normal ($728 \pm$ S.D. 140 mg/100 ml). Clinically, these children show tendon xanthomas, corneal arcus, xanthelasma, and arthritis. Both erythrocyte sedimentation rate and plasma fibrinogen are elevated. Atherosclerosis, once it begins, takes a galloping course, the mean age at death being 21 years (range 13–37).

The heterozygote is much more difficult to identify. Serum cholesterol elevation in cord blood above 100 mg is suggestive. In older children and adults there is a significant overlap between heterozygotes and so-called normal individuals who consume high-fat diets. In the heterozygote, dietary management is the mainstay of treatment. Placing these patients on the "prudent diet" recommended by the American Heart Association will often keep cholesterol levels between 200 and 250 mg/100 ml. As age advances, however, cholesterol levels begin to creep up and dietary management becomes less effective.

Charles J. Glueck, associate professor of medicine and pediatrics at the University of Cincinnati College of Medicine, discussed hyperlipidemia further. He first pointed out that there is mounting concern that the apparent progression from fatty streak to fibrous plaques and then to full-fledged atheromatous plaques is an indication that coronary heart disease may begin in childhood. He noted also that a great number of children and young adults have elevated levels of serum cholesterol. For example, in one study 6 to 7% of the schoolchildren had levels above 220 mg percent. In another study, 14% of the children between the ages of 12 and 15 had cholesterol levels greater than 260 mg percent. Dr. Glueck feels, therefore, that one approach to the primary prevention of cardiovascular disease might be to identify children with elevated levels of cholesterol and triglyceride, or both, and to do whatever one can to treat them. The two most common hyperlipidemias in children are hypercholesterolemia, with a primary elevation of cholesterol and beta lipoprotein of cholesterol (LDL), and hypertriglyceridemia, with a primary elevation of triglycerides and very low density lipoprotein cholesterol (VLDL). In a small number of children, cholesterol, triglycerides, LDL, and VLDL are all elevated.

Dr. Glueck's studies, based on screening 1800 newborns, suggest a frequency for familial hypercholesterolemia of about 0.9%. Those 0.9% also have elevated levels of cholesterol at age 1 year. Screening later in childhood makes it difficult to separate children with familial hypercholesterolemia from those with the diet-induced form. Hypertriglyceridemia in childhood cannot be diagnosed from cord blood. If there is a family history of this condition, repeated serum levels should be taken. Since these diseases are transmitted as autosomal dominants, it is important to carry out a complete family screening if an adult member of the family has any form of hyperlipidemia. A second approach, which has identified a high percentage of affected children, has been to screen all members of a family in which either parent had a coronary occlusion before age 50.

Finally, if resources will allow, all newborns and schoolchildren might be screened.

Experience indicates that among school-age children there are two to three hypercholesterolemics whose families have no evidence of hypercholesterolemia for every one whose family does. In the former cases, dietary history often demonstrates a cholesterol intake of 600 to 1200 mg/day and an average polyunsaturated/saturated ratio of about 0.3:0.4. This is in contrast to an average intake of 400 to 600 mg/day and an average ratio of 0.2:0.5 among American children. A prudent low-cholesterol diet, containing approximately 200 mg of cholesterol and a polyunsaturate/saturate ratio of 1.5:1, will almost always normalize the cholesterol levels of affected children. Dietary therapy for children with familial hypercholesterolemia is begun at 1 year, using a modification of the National Institutes of Health type 2 diet. On this diet, which contains less than 200 mg of cholesterol and a P/S ratio of 1.5:1, the cholesterol level in from 60 to 80% of children will drop to normal. As the children get older, however, fewer and fewer will respond to this type of dietary management. Hypertriglyceridemia in children is relatively easy to treat. First and foremost is weight reduction in those who are obese. This treatment will usually reduce serum triglyceride levels to normal. If, however, they remain elevated, a National Heart Institute type 4 diet (a balanced proportion of calories, 20% as protein, 40% as fat, and 40% as carbohydrate and moderately rich in polyunsaturates) is effective in maintaining normal triglyceride levels. Extrapolating from primate studies, Dr. Glueck expressed the hope that keeping plasma cholesterol or triglycerides normal in children, whether their disease is familial or acquired, may limit the formation of irreversible atherosclerotic plaques.

Prevention of coronary artery disease in adults by tackling obesity in childhood was the major theme of Dr. Glenn Friedman, a practicing pediatrician on the faculty of the University of Arizona. He reminded the audience that there are five major factors that predispose to coronary heart disease: hypercholesterolemia, hypertension, cigarette smoking, obesity, and sedentary living. Dr. Friedman reasoned that "since the above five risk factors probably are harmful and since they each have been related to our cardiovascular epidemic as well as to other disease processes, it would seem reasonable to reduce or prevent these factors from developing in the child and his parents without either producing anxiety or decreasing the joy of living." He argued that the time to begin prevention is in childhood because that is when patterns of living that lead to risk patterns begin. Atherosclerosis does develop in the pediatric age group and may be reversible in this age group. Finally, by reducing developing risk factors in the child, parents' risk factors may also be reduced.

Putting this philosophy into practice, Dr. Friedman has helped to organize two screening intervention programs in Arizona. In his office some 3400 middle-class children have been tested for serum cholesterol, blood pressure, subcutaneous fat, and maximal endurance on the bicycle ergometer. Their histories, which include details of milk consumption and exercise, have been recorded. Parents too were measured for total cholesterol, blood pressure, and subcutaneous fat. Their family histories of cardiovascular disease were taken, and notations were made on their use of tobacco and indulgence in exercise. The tests on the children were begun at the age of 1 month and continued at regular intervals, even on healthy children. A similar program, sponsored by the state health department, is under way in certain rural areas of Arizona.

When Dr. Friedman spots a child he considers to be at risk, he takes the following steps in the following manner. By reporting to the parents all test results in relation to "desirable levels" he motivates them to promote changes; he reinforces various segments of the program with pamphlets and visual aids; one evening a month he holds a slide presentation which is open to the community; last, he has the services of a nutritionist in his office.

Dr. Friedman has developed an alternative to the low-fat, low-cholesterol diet because, he said, he has found it difficult to persuade his patients to adhere to it for very long. He controls the intake of cholesterol by limiting the protein intake to the recommended dietary allowances. Since protein-rich animal products are also usually high in cholesterol and saturated fat, he creates what is, in effect, a cholesterol quantity-exchange diet pegged to the recommended protein allowance. If the protein recommendations are not exceeded, it is difficult for the patient to get too much fat or cholesterol in the diet. In addition to these dietary manipulations, a parent with hypertension is referred for medical help, smoking is discouraged, and parents are encouraged to lose weight, when appropriate, and to increase their exercise. Children who are obese are managed by dietary means through parental counciling. Dr. Friedman concluded by observing that "we are dealing with an iceberg. The disease process and the risk factors have their inception in the pediatric age group, where there is presently no significant screening or intervention. It is only when the problem emerges from the sea with the onset of a coronary or a stroke that we seem to get concerned. By then it is too late. We must start earlier."

From the discussions of obesity and hyperlipidemia in the young, we turned our attention to therapy for childhood obesity. This aspect has drawn more and more interest as the diet craze has slowly filtered down from our weight-conscious adult society to the children in our midst.

Three specific approaches to therapy were discussed. These were dietary management, the use of hormones in obesity, and psychological management of the fat child.

Jerome Knittle, professor of pediatrics at Mount Sinai Medical School in New York City, led off with his observations about various aspects of the dietary management of childhood obesity. Animal studies had shown, he said, that only when dietary management began early in life could the number of fat cells be altered. His statement was based on his studies of both normal and obese children. He showed that some obese children had acquired the adult number of fat cells by the time they were 3 years old. Prognosis in such cases is quite dark. Children who have too many adipocytes for their age, but still have fewer than the normal adult number, have a better chance to avoid adult obesity. However, the aim is to slow down the rate of adipocyte division while maintaining normal, or at least near normal, growth. Weight reduction is not advocated for such patients. Dr. Knittle took the position that the aim of restricting the diet is to have the child maintain his weight but "grow out of his obesity."

Hormones have very little, if any, place in the treatment of childhood obesity, according to Richard Rivlin, associate professor in the department of medicine of Columbia University's College of Physicians and Surgeons and the Institute of Human Nutrition. He noted that although certain workers have claimed success with chorionic gonadotropin, the results of controlled studies are, at best, inconclusive. Thyroid hormone produces weight loss, but only while it is being taken. It depletes nitrogen and calcium stores, but causes relatively little loss of body fat. The cardiovascular effects of thyroid hormone may constitute a risk, and its known effect on skeletal growth is an even greater hazard in childhood. Thus the indiscriminate use of thyroid hormone is to be discouraged. Although its use is not practical, human growth hormone has certain attractive features for the treatment of obesity. It mobilizes body fat and promotes nitrogen retention. However, it is recommended only for children who are deficient in growth hormone. At present, then, there is no hormonal agent that can be used safely and effectively to treat childhood obesity.

Dr. Henry Jordan from the department of psychiatry of the University of Pennsylvania School of Medicine in Philadelphia approaches childhood obesity as a matter requiring behavioral modification. The initial phase of treatment focuses on analyzing behavior and keeping accurate records to determine what behavior is maladaptive. Once that has been done, emphasis is placed on gradual changes in behavior, rather than on weight loss per se. This approach was tried on overweight children, and an average weight loss of 6.2 pounds in 10 weeks was achieved. Follow-up was incomplete but that fact alone served to emphasize the need for physicians to develop techniques that would gradually shift the responsibility for treatment from the therapist to the parents and children. Thus, although much more research in this area is needed, the behavior-modification approach seems to offer promise as a useful therapeutic tool in the treatment of childhood obesity.

Drs. Marci Greenwood and Patricia Johnson discuss the behavioral characteristics involved in the genesis and maintenance of obesity. They cite experiments with animals in which the neural control of appetite is localized and describe these experiments and their implications in obesity. They critically review the various theories about the human drive to eat. In addition they examine the behavioral characteristics involved in controlling activity.

As can be noted from the chapters that follow, it is apparent that a great deal is now known about childhood obesity, its causes, and present methods of treatment. Perhaps most important is the fact that childhood obesity is now recognized as a significant health hazard; to eradicate it the medical community, the nutrition community, and concerned parents must be mobilized. We must now move ahead from this knowledge to the much more difficult problem of preventing this progression, which is of such major importance in acquiring our goal of healthier and happier adults.

PART 1

Cellular Changes

1

Cell Number and Size as a Determinant of Subsequent Obesity

JULES HIRSCH, M.D.

Rockefeller University, New York, New York

Perhaps the most universally recognized fact about obesity is the intractability of this disorder and thus the frequent failure of treatment, whether by diet, drugs, or psychotherapy. In an effort to explain this phenomenon, the members of my laboratory and I have studied obesity by carefully observing subjects who had lost weight to "normal" as the result of caloric restriction during a long hospitalization. We were most concerned with finding what abnormality tended to propel them back to their previous obese weight. A variety of potentially interesting behavioral disorders have been found in such reduced subjects (1), but another intriguing finding has been a sharp change in the morphology of adipose tissue, suggesting that cell number remained constant during weight reduction and only cell size had changed. Many of these previously obese subjects persisted in having an excessive number of unusually small adipocytes when compared with the usual morphologic findings of control subjects who had never been obese.

These findings have led to the hypothesis that obesity may be accompanied by an excessive number of adipocytes, possibly brought about by excess feeding in infancy and childhood, and that the excessive number of adipocytes remains constant and in some way causes a drive for main-

Supported by research grants 03719 and 02761 from the National Institutes of Health.

taining the obese state. Such an hypothesis demands that there be some clear link between the state of cell filling or cell number and the overall energy metabolism of the subject, in terms of either feeding behavior or energy loss. This link between adipose tissue and the central nervous system remains totally speculative. Nevertheless, this hypothesis has led to considerable recent interest in examining adipose tissue morphology in both man and animals. These speculations have also been criticized (2,3,4). In this chapter we examine critically the connection between adipose cellularity and obesity and suggest further studies that may lead to either a strengthening or a rejection of these ideas.

Every organ grows and matures by some combination of cellular enlargement and cell replication and, in general, cell replication is a forerunner of cellular enlargement. In some organs the ability to continue growth by further cell replication is lost early in life (e.g., brain), whereas in other tissues growth and renewal by cell replication and by enlargement of cells continues uninterrupted throughout life (e.g., liver). Presumably, the situation with adipose tissue is somewhere between these two extremes. The idea that alterations in cellularity are induced by inborn differences or early nutritional experiences has been an active area of exploration, particularly in brain structure and function. Thus the concept that similar considerations could be of interest in adipose tissue development and function is by no means "bizarre in biologic affairs" as one critic has suggested (4). But all would seem to depend on the nature of adipose tissue growth and its metabolic consequences.

During recent years, fairly rapid and accurate methods have become available for the sizing and counting of human and animal adipocytes (5). These methods share a common fault; namely, only cells with some lipid content can be identified and counted. Indeed, the presence of lipid is the sole identifying characteristic of the adipocyte. Cells with extremely small amounts of stored fat, less than 25 μ in diameter and generally fewer than 1% of the adipocytes seen microscopically in adipose tissue, are lost to these methods. Thus cells essentially devoid of lipid that may be destined to store lipid at some later date and might be designated as preadipocytes cannot be counted. But given these shortcomings, it is worth examining the findings to date.

ADIPOSE CELLULARITY IN OBESE MAN

Several hundred obese subjects have been submitted to a careful examination of adipocyte size and simultaneous estimation of total adipocyte number in my own laboratory as well as in the studies of Bjorntorp and colleagues (6) in Sweden and Salans and colleagues (7) in this country. There is unanimity that the vast majority of obese subjects have some adipocyte enlargement. But in many instances and particularly in the massively obese there is a startling increase in cell number as well. This elevation of cell number does not change appreciably with weight reduction, although at times cells shrink to such a degree with extreme weight reduction that they are lost in the counting and sizing procedures. It seems evident, furthermore, that the increased adipocyte number is not gradually rectified over time. Both in the persistently obese state and in the weight-reduced state, the cell number, at least in adult man, is unchanging. These interesting findings have prompted a careful analysis of the cellular development of adipose tissue in various animal strains.

DEVELOPMENT OF CELLULARITY IN ANIMAL ADIPOSE TISSUE

Adipose tissue as studied in the rat (8) develops early by a pattern of combined hyperplasia and hypertrophy, gradually changing to growth exclusively by enlargement of cells with no further change in cell number. The establishment of adult cell number occurs at different times in epididymal, retroperitoneal, or subcutaneous depots, but in all sites further or new appearance of cells ceases by 10 to 14 weeks of age. Neither a reduction in adipose tissue mass by acute starvation or more chronic underfeeding nor an enlargement of the depot by overfeeding produces any change in cell number, although cell size remains extremely elastic (8).

EXPERIMENTAL OBESITY IN MAN AND ANIMALS

Two further pieces of evidence in support of the early establishment and fixed nature of cell number come from studies of experimental obesity. In man, Sims and his colleagues (9) have shown that purposely overfed adult volunteers can be transiently made moderately obese. When this type of experimental obesity occurs, there is exclusively an enlargement of cells, as though the obesity occurring in this manner cannot alter a basically fixed cell number that was established prior to the onset of obesity. Hence this situation is in contrast to spontaneously occurring obesity in man in which cell number is often elevated. The second piece of evidence is the finding that rats and mice made obese as adults either by electrolytic ablation of hypothalamic food intake control areas or by the administration of gold thioglucose (which likewise is believed to interfere with the central nervous system control of food intake) all develop mammoth enlargement of adipose depots, but exclusively by cell enlargement with no significant change in a fixed cell number. It thus becomes of considerable interest to ascertain what influences can be found to alter cell number.

EARLY NUTRITIONAL INFLUENCES AND ADIPOSE CELLULARITY

In reviewing their data on cellularity in quite markedly obese human subjects, Salans, et al. (7) found that the hyperplastic members of their group showed a high incidence of obesity beginning in childhood. This suggests, but by no means proves, that some factors acting in early childhood, perhaps overnutrition, can be responsible for setting cell number at a high and permanently fixed level. Some earlier animal work lends further plausibility to this idea.

Knittle and I (10) showed that when infant rats are stunted in growth by undernutrition in the first 3 weeks of life, it is possible to create a permanent decrease in both adipocyte number and size when compared with infant rats reared under more usual or optimal conditions. These changes persist even though all animals have ad libitum access to food beginning at weaning or at roughly 3 weeks of age. After 3 weeks of age it is difficult if not impossible to make similar permanent alterations in adipose cellularity. This is somewhat surprising since cells continue to appear in the cell adipose depots of the rat for several weeks following weaning. If these experiments can be considered evidence of the early fixation of cell number, then it appears that this biologic decision is made very early when cells are continuing to fill with triglyceride and make their appearance as mature adipocytes.

Although all of the above lines of inquiry lend support to the hypothesis that a fixed cell number, which can be set at some higher level, is arrived at early in life and that such an increase is generative of adult obesity, some very serious criticisms can be and have been (2,3,4) leveled at this work. To begin with, there may be a turnover of mature adipocytes such that some cells disappear and are replaced by newly maturing "preadipocytes." Thus the fixed-number concept may not imply a final cellular event occurring in infancy, but rather some control of total adipose mass, similar for example to the delicate control of erythrocyte mass in which erythopoietin and other factors modulate the total cellular mass, yet the cells are in continuous and rapid turnover.

This possibility has been studied initially by Hollenberg and his associates (11) and also in my laboratory by Greenwood (12). It has been shown that the administration of relatively large doses of tritiated thymidine to the rat leads to essentially no immediate incorporation into mature adipocytes. Some days after the injection, however, a minute amount of isotopic label can be found in the DNA of adipocytes. This is most likely evidence for the formation of labeled DNA in a precursor cell that can be termed a preadipocyte and then its filling with lipid over some days, after which it can be identified as an adipocyte, harvested, and studied. When Greenwood and I attempted to measure the degree to which such newly synthesized preadipocytes fill and are added to the mature adipocyte pool, we found that in older animals at roughly 5 months of age there was no measurable addition of new cells. Thus, from such studies, the pool of mature adipocytes can be considered to be inert in terms of cellular turnover and renewal.

We were also interested in determining the ages at which preadipocytes can form and be added to the pool of mature adipocytes. For this purpose, tritiated thymidine was administered to large numbers of rats at various times from earliest infancy onward. Groups of animals were killed at various time intervals following injection to determine the rate at which labeled DNA was added to the adipocyte pool. The data obtained are not always unambiguous because of some contamination of stromal, nonadipocyte elements which have vastly more radioactivity than adipocytes. But the likeliest interpretation strongly suggests the following. Until weaning there is a simultaneous formation of many preadipocytes along with filling of a fraction of these adipocytes to give an increasing number of mature adipocytes. Shortly after weaning, or at 3 to 4 weeks of life, the formation of new preadipocytes tapers off quickly and all newly formed mature adipocytes result from the filling of preadipocytes formed earlier.

Since some of the criticism of the adipose cellularity hypothesis and obesity stems from the notion that there may be small adipocytes or preadipocyltes that can fill at any time in adult life, these experiments would seem to be a further piece of evidence in favor of the early and final formation of adipocytes and their precursors. Interestingly, the finding that most precursor cells are formed by the time of weaning may serve as an explanation for why postweaning nutritional influences have so little permanent effect on rat adipose cell number, even though mature adipocytes are continuing to appear at this early time of life.

A confounding and troubling piece of evidence that speaks against these theories is the frequently found obese human who by medical history has become obese as an adult and yet has an excessive number of adipocytes. Were the cells always there in some precursor form or do these individuals have the ability to form adipocytes even in adult life? No clear answer is at hand.

Two future lines of investigation would seem to be particularly helpful in evaluating to what degree adipose cellularity is a determinant of obesity.

1. Some technique for distinguishing among the many cellular types that constitute the supportive stroma of adipose tissue and establishing which cell is a potential or actual preadipocyte would be most useful. Perhaps by enzyme markers or by some technique of special histochemistry one might identify and number these important cells. No matter how obese an infant may be, it is clear that most of the mature cellular mass of adipocytes must develop at some later age. Are the precursor cells identifiable and, if so, at what age do they appear? The answers to these questions would help unscramble present data on human adipose cellularity, which at best shows only some relationship between age of onset of obesity and cell number, but not the hard and fixed correlation that one would need to separate genetic factors, early nutrition, and other influences on adipose cellularity and establish their meaning in the genesis of adult human obesity.

2. Since the concept of a fixed cell number has been dubbed a "fatalistic" concept it is somehow implied that cell number and its fixed state is forever a call to the central nervous system to alter feeding behavior or perhaps energy metabolism in such a way as to keep these cells filled with lipid. Such ideas necessitate a signal from adipose tissue cells to brain. Although there has been a great deal of recent speculation about brain "set points" and an even older speculation about long-term regulators of food intake, no clear and defined signals have been described. Models of food-intake control have been elaborated (13), which can be most intriguing if an adipose signal is assumed, but without laboratory evidence the meaning of adipose cellularity in such terms remains unknown.

There is abundant literature describing the metabolic intricacies of adipose tissue and it is also well known that some significant biochemical parameters, such as the sensitivity of the tissue to hormone action, are to some degree a function of cell size and cell number, but how these findings can be translated into a centrally received signal is unknown. Thus, this remains a most significant area of research, for without such a signal the meaning of adipose cellularity in human obesity could be relegated to an interesting and associated finding, but not one which can in any way be considered a determinant of obesity.

Whatever the final verdict may be, the above speculations and findings concerning adipose cellularity have at least had the advantage of opening one line of investigation that might be experimentally validated. Other speculations on obesity, which are concerned with the "lack of self-control" of the obese or with general theories of the social and economic pressures wrought by the availability of foodstuffs, seem less likely to be validated in controlled, laboratory-based studies.

REFERENCES

1. J. Grinker and J. Hirsch, Ciba Foundation Symposium 8 (new series). Amsterdam: ASP, 1972, p. 349.

2. E. M. Widdowson and W. T. Shaw, Lancet 1: 905 (1973).

3. M. Ashwell and J. S. Garrow, Lancet 1: 1036 (1973).

4. G. V. Mann, N. Engl. J. Med. 291: 226 (1974).

5. J. Hirsch and E. Gallian, J. Lipid Res. 9: 110 (1968).

6. P. Bjorntorp and L. Sjostrom, Metabolism 20: 703 (1971).

7. L. B. Salans, S. W. Cushman, and R. E. Weismann, J. Clin. Invest. 52: 929 (1973).

8. J. Hirsch and P. W. Han, J. Lipid Res. 10: 77 (1969).

9. E. A. H. Sims, R. F. Goldman, C. M. Gluck, E. S. Horton, P. C. Kelleher, and D. W. Rowe, Trans. Assn. Am. Physicians 81: 153 (1968).

10. J. L. Knittle and J. Hirsch, J. Clin. Invest. 47: 2091 (1961).

11. C. H. Hollenberg and A. Vost, J. Clin. Invest. 47: 2485 (1968).

12. M. R. C. Greenwood and J. Hirsch, J. Lipid Res. 15: 474 (1974).

13. J. Hirsch, Adv. Psychosom. Med. 7: 229 (1972).

2

Growth, Body Composition, and Development of Obese and Lean Children

STANLEY M. GARN, M.D.

with

DIANE C. CLARK and KENNETH E. GUIRE

Center for Human Growth and Development and The Human Nutrition Program, School of Public Health, University of Michigan, Ann Arbor, Michigan.

Over the past 20 years we have become concerned with both extremes of fatness, in infants, in children, and beyond. The least degrees of fatness have attracted our attention in areas where malnutrition is chronic, or where acute malnutrition exists, or where protein-calorie malnutrition occurs. Overly lean children are sick more often, more likely to die, they are apt to become size-reduced adults, and they may present problems of learning along with obvious problems of growing.

The higher levels of fatness have attracted attention more recently as a by-product of our concern with adult obesity. We no longer value high levels of weight gain during infancy, pudgy babies with buffalo necks, or infant giants. There is the often-expressed fear that the fat baby is on a programmed path to adult obesity, atherosclerosis, and early demise from cardiovascular-renal disorders.

But we know little of childhood obesity, including its very measurement and definition. We cannot apply overly simple overweight standards when weight is so related to size and rather imperfectly related to measured fatness. There is the problem of defining obesity, when the level of fatness varies with socioeconomic status, and may not be the same in boys and girls of different ancestral origins even at the same economic levels.

We have little direct information on the growth of fat infants and children as compared with those who are lean, or their body composition, or their hematology, or their lipid levels. And despite some semilongitudinal epidemiologic data on the adult characteristics of older children differing in relative weight, we do not have lifelong human models that tell us (even retrospectively) of the prospective future of fat infants and children.

In this chapter we attempt to clarify, if not resolve, some of these problems. We discuss, first, the quantitative definition of obesity and leanness in infants and children; second, some of the problems of definition that socioeconomic differences bring about; and third, some growth-related implications of fatness and leanness in infants and children. Fourth, we consider fatness-related differences in body composition and in hematological status; and finally (or fifth), the question of whether fat babies inevitably turn out to be obese adults.

The human model is appropriate here because it introduces some complications that are so far lacking in laboratory studies of fatness. If fatness level is positively correlated with the level of affluence in prepubertal girls, yet negatively related with affluence in girls grown up, then we cannot be so sure that fatness is early imprinted at the cellular level, or that it is truly irreversible. And if lean, impoverished girls become fat, impoverished women, then we may have to go back to the rat cage for a better experimental design.

MEASURING OBESITY AND LEANNESS

Though concerned with obesity, that is, excessive fatness, or corpulence in the older terminology (3), most investigators have actually employed relative weight or relative overweight in the absence of direct measures of fatness. A few, more sophisticated, have considered the possibility of using relative weight or relative overweight (12) for height, in order to grant size some measure of correction. Of course, relative weight (actual weight divided by some standard weight) is not mathematically different from actual weight, being weight divided by a constant. And standard weight, as derived from some table, is not necessarily ideal weight, and it ignores individual differences in the size of the fat-free weight (FFW). But the question is how do relative weight, relative overweight, and percentage overweight compare with measured fatness in infants, in children, and even later.

To answer this question we have taken the traditional and accepted value of 20% overweight (120% of standard weight) in a very large series of people, from infancy through old age. Then we have investigated the relative overweight of the obese individuals, defining as obese those individuals at or above the eighty-fifth percentile for measured triceps fatness. The question is how the relative weight of such obese infants, children, and adolescents matches the traditional 20% overweight line.

The results, simply graphed in Fig. 1, are more than interesting. They show that for adult women the relative weight of the obese group (>eighty-fifth fatness percentile) reasonably approximates the 20% overweight line, *for that group*. For adolescents, however, the obese group falls above the 20% overweight line, and for infants and children, the measured obese fall well below the 20% overweight level. Clearly a single overweight level does not define obesity equally well in infants, in preschool children, in school-age girls, and in adolescents alike.

We have also explored the correlations between measured fatness (using the compressed double triceps fat fold) and relative weight for age and also relative weight for both age and standing height. Again the results, expressed in Table 1, are interested indeed. For infants relative weight is rather poorly related to measured fatness—about 0.20. With increasing age, the correlations get higher, peaking above 0.7 in adolescent girls. Corrections for size, using partial correlations, are scarcely better. The evidence indicates that for 900 children in the 1 to 3 year age group, relative weight (or relative weight for height) is hardly appropriate as a measure of fatness or corpulence. It gets better for 1388 preschool

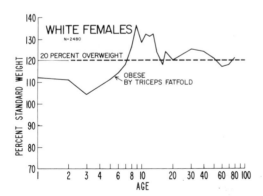

Figure 1. Relative weight, expressed as a percent of standard weight (ordinate), of children and adults defined as obese by the triceps fat fold. Adults at or beyond the eighty-fifth percentile for the triceps fat fold reasonably approximate the 20% overweight level (dashed line), whereas equally obese infants and early school-age children are well below the 20% overweight level.

Table 1   Comparison of Fat-fold Thickness and Relative Weight as a Measure of Fatness

		Fat Fold versus Relative Weight				
		Boys			Girls	
Age	N	r versus Relative Weight	r versus Relative Weight/Height[a]	N	r versus Relative Weight	r versus Relative Weight/Height[a]
1	129	0.11	0.08	157	0.40	0.44
2	164	0.06	0.15	156	0.25	0.17
3	200	0.09	0.08	154	0.26	0.35
4	201	0.37	0.47	210	0.37	0.42
5	254	0.55	0.55	227	0.25	0.29
6	252	0.42	0.45	244	0.43	0.45
7	304	0.52	0.51	263	0.54	0.54
8	289	0.65	0.65	255	0.60	0.62
9	278	0.59	0.59	272	0.27	0.19
10	308	0.65	0.69	268	0.63	0.67
11	285	0.72	0.71	261	0.67	0.69
12	286	0.66	0.73	260	0.65	0.74
13	256	0.52	0.71	223	0.73	0.80
14	201	0.45	0.64	180	0.76	0.78
15	177	0.51	0.67	191	0.67	0.72
16	158	0.59	0.71	182	0.62	0.66
17	137	0.55	0.62	138	0.72	0.74

[a] Partial correlation $(r_{12.3})$ fat fold versus relative weight corrected for height.

boys and girls. But even in 4000 boys and girls in the primary-school age range, relative weight (or relative weight corrected for height) is no great measure of fatness or leanness.

Accordingly we have defined obesity and leanness entirely in terms of the measured triceps fat folds, for which we have data on some 20,000 people of European ancestry (and an equal number of African and Mexican-American derivation). We have selected, with computer assistance, an obese group (at or above the eighty-fifth percentile for the triceps fat fold for age and sex). We have also selected a lean group (at or below the fifteenth percentile for triceps fatness for age and sex). The cutoff values for the triceps fat fold, representing the eighty-fifth percentile (obese) and the fifteenth percentile (lean) are detailed in Table 2, for several reasons. First, we want to define the cutoff levels we have used, based on age-sex distributions. Second, we want to make them available to other workers, who may want to extend these studies. Third, we want to point out the fatness of the obese (so defined) relative to that of the

Table 2   Fifteenth and Eighty-fifth Percentile Cutoff Values for Lean and Obese Children

		Males					Females		
		Obese	Lean	Ratio			Obese	Lean	Ratio
	Total	85th	15th	Obese/	Total		85th	15th	Obese/
Age	N	Percentile	Percentile	Lean	N		Percentile	Percentile	Lean
1	126	9.0	6.0	1.50	—		—	—	—
2	163	13.0	7.0	1.86	47		12.0	5.0	2.40
3	175	13.0	7.0	1.86	156		12.0	7.0	1.71
4	177	12.0	6.0	2.00	147		12.0	7.0	1.71
5	229	12.0	6.0	2.00	145		12.0	7.0	1.71
6	224	12.0	6.0	2.00	190		13.0	7.0	1.86
7	278	12.0	6.0	2.00	210		14.0	7.0	2.00
8	271	12.0	6.0	2.00	224		12.0	7.0	1.71
9	258	15.0	6.0	2.50	241		14.0	7.0	2.00
10	279	15.0	6.0	2.50	231		15.0	7.0	2.14
11	259	17.0	7.0	2.43	254		18.0	8.0	2.25
12	252	19.0	7.0	2.71	247		20.0	8.0	2.50
13	245	18.0	7.0	2.57	241		20.0	8.0	2.50
14	170	18.0	6.0	3.00	229		20.0	9.0	2.22
15	167	20.0	6.0	3.33	202		22.0	9.0	2.44
16	131	19.0	5.0	3.80	163		23.0	10.0	2.30
17	120	14.0	5.0	2.80	169		23.0	11.0	2.09

[a] All values to the nearest whole millimeter consistent with the readout of the fat-fold caliper.

lean. For boys, the cutoff values for the obese are twice that of the lean, through age 8, and three times so in later adolescence. For girls, despite their greater absolute fatness at all ages, the obese cutoffs (>eighty-fifth percentile) are not much more than 2.5 times as fat as the lean cutoffs (<fifteenth percentile). This difference we may remember, later in this chapter.

Of course the fat fold cutoff values given in Table 2 are only the lower limits of leanness. The *groups* so defined as obese and as lean are fatter still, and leaner still, respectively. So it is useful, as in Table 3, to compare the fatness of the obese group and that of the lean group. The results are even more impressive and more important to the investigative sections that follow.

As a group, the *obese* boys are 2 to 5 times as fat as the lean, depending upon age. As a group, the *obese* girls are 2.0 to 3.5 times as fat as the lean, depending upon age. These generalized values should be held in mind when we later compare the growth, nutrition, and body composition of obese infants and children with their lean age-peers. If we are con-

Table 3   Comparative Fatness of Obese and Lean Boys and Girls

Age	Male Fatness Medians[a]			Female Fatness Medians[a]		
	Obese (mm)	Lean (mm)	Ratio Obese/Lean	Obese (mm)	Lean (mm)	Ratio Obese/Lean
1	14.0	6.0	2.33	—	—	—
2	14.0	6.0	2.33	13.0	5.0	2.60
3	14.0	6.0	2.33	14.0	6.0	2.33
4	13.0	6.0	2.17	14.0	7.0	2.00
5	13.0	5.0	2.60	13.0	6.0	2.17
6	14.0	5.0	2.80	14.0	6.0	2.33
7	14.0	5.0	2.80	15.0	6.0	2.50
8	15.0	5.0	3.00	14.0	6.0	2.33
9	18.0	5.0	3.60	16.0	6.0	2.67
10	19.0	5.0	3.80	17.0	6.0	2.83
11	20.0	6.0	3.33	23.0	7.0	3.29
12	23.0	6.0	3.83	23.0	7.0	3.29
13	22.0	7.0	3.14	24.0	7.0	3.43
14	20.0	5.0	4.00	24.0	7.0	3.43
15	25.0	5.0	5.00	26.0	7.0	3.71
16	24.0	4.0	6.00	27.0	8.0	3.38
17	18.0	4.0	4.50	28.0	9.0	3.11

[a] Triceps fat-fold values for the obese and lean as defined by the cutoff values given in Table 2.

cerned, as we are here, with the developmental, gravimetric, and biochemical concomitants of obesity and leanness, we need to know how much fatter the obese are than the measured lean.

PHYSICAL AND BIOCHEMICAL DEVELOPMENT OF OBESE AND LEAN CHILDREN

Despite the interest in obesity on the one hand and leanness on the other, there have been few studies of the metric, skeletal, and biochemical development of obese and lean boys and girls. Such few studies as we have do indicate statural and skeletal advancement in obese children in both Scandinavia (11) and England (14), consistent with the "supernutrition" hypothesis, and of "hyperpituitarism due to hyperphagia." In the United States we have previously explored the relationship between radiogrammetric fat-shadow measurements and both size and skeletal development, such that the fatter are taller and skeletally advanced (6,7). These generalizations apply to school-age children and into adolescence.

Since fatness during the first year of life peaks and then declines consistent with an abrupt increase in the fat-free weight, some fat 1-year-olds may be developmentally younger than their chronologic age, complicating the problem of generalizations prior to the age of walking.

Among our subjects (13) obese boys and girls are taller than their lean age-peers from at least the second year on (5). At age 2 the difference is of the order of 4 cm (as shown in Table 4) and this difference in standing height increases to approximately 5 cm at age 12. The difference in size between obese and lean boys and girls is approximately 1 standard deviation (σ). By way of comparison, the weight difference (in kg) between

Table 4   Height, Weight, Hemoglobin, and Vitamin C in Obese and Lean Children

Age	Weight kg		Height cm		Hemoglobin (gm/100 ml)		Ascorbic Acid (mg/100 ml)	
	Obese	Lean	Obese	Lean	Obese	Lean	Obese	Lean
				Males				
1	—	—	—	—	—	—	—	—
2	13.0	11.6	86.6	82.6	12.2	11.4	0.30	0.54
3	15.8	14.2	96.4	94.3	11.7	12.1	1.34	1.04
4	17.7	15.6	101.9	102.1	12.7	12.0	0.83	0.44
5	21.1	17.5	111.7	107.3	12.5	12.3	0.86	0.50
6	22.0	19.7	116.0	113.5	12.6	12.4	1.06	0.77
7	25.7	21.3	123.8	119.4	12.7	12.6	0.86	0.64
8	29.6	23.3	129.6	123.3	13.0	12.6	0.73	0.84
9	33.8	26.0	133.8	130.5	13.3	12.8	0.93	0.83
10	39.8	27.7	137.6	134.7	13.3	12.8	0.69	0.86
11	47.5	30.7	146.8	139.1	13.1	13.1	0.85	0.91
12	52.7	33.5	149.9	144.3	13.5	13.1	0.69	0.85
				Females				
1	—	—	—	—	—	—	—	—
2	13.2	11.8	88.0	84.0	11.9	11.9	1.12	1.21
3	13.9	12.7	90.7	92.0	11.5	12.1	0.37	0.79
4	16.5	14.0	101.7	98.4	12.3	12.1	1.57	0.63
5	19.2	16.7	106.1	105.4	12.5	12.3	1.21	0.71
6	21.4	18.2	114.9	111.8	12.3	12.3	0.91	0.68
7	26.1	20.4	122.7	117.1	12.8	12.7	1.25	0.40
8	30.4	22.2	126.2	123.8	13.1	12.8	0.81	0.84
9	36.6	24.9	135.7	129.0	13.4	12.8	0.72	0.97
10	40.1	28.5	139.7	135.4	13.2	12.5	0.58	0.74
11	50.4	29.8	145.8	138.4	13.4	12.7	0.79	0.83
12	53.8	35.1	151.1	146.4	13.4	12.9	0.62	0.87

[a] Obese and lean groups as in Table 3.

obese and lean boys and girls increases from less than 2 kg at the second year to nearly 20 kg at age 12, as detailed in Table 4.

We have explored, in considerable detail, the relationship between fat thickness (mm) and growth in size (cm), setting up a series of fatness intervals as in Fig. 2. The results are quite consistent in both sexes. If we take the triceps double fat fold into consideration, four fatness levels (in mm) show systematically different levels of size attainment, age by age, and it is clear that in both sexes the fatter children are the taller as they grow (Δ size has a fairly linear relationship to Δ fat). This statement specifically applies within populations, though it may also be applicable between related populations.

In a general way, obese boys and girls have higher hemoglobin levels than do lean boys and girls, as also shown in Table 4, and they have higher hematocrits too. Taken the other way, boys and girls with high hemoglobin levels (>eighty-fifth percentile for age and sex) tend to be fatter and those with low hemoglobin levels tend to be leaner (9). This generalization applies at the adult level as well. Obese individuals, we find, tend to have relative polycythemia.

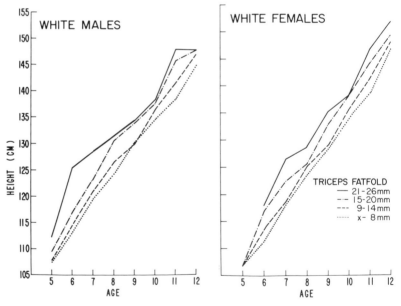

Figure 2. Growth in stature (standing height) at four levels of fatness, in prepubertal white boys and girls. For four different levels of fatness, growth rates and size attainment are systematically different, with the fattest boys and girls the tallest at all ages shown (5).

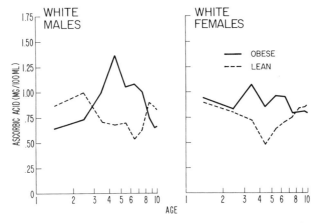

Figure 3. Serum ascorbic acid levels in obese boys and girls (heavy line) and lean boys and girls (dashed line). In general, the obese children (the upper 15% for triceps fatness) of both sexes tend to have higher serum ascorbic acid levels, just as they have higher hemoglobin levels (gm/100 cc) and higher hematocrits, have higher levels of vitamin A, and are taller and advanced in skeletal and sexual maturation.

We have also explored various serum and urinary vitamin levels in the obese and lean boys and girls described in Tables 2 to 4. The obese children do tend to have higher levels of vitamins A and C (Fig. 3) and several of the B vitamins, but the relationships between fatness and serum and urinary vitamins are not nearly as impressive as the relationships between income level and the same serum and urinary vitamins.

As a safe generalization, the obese boys and girls (age 2 to 12) are taller than the lean, as shown in Table 4 and Fig. 2. They are, of course, much heavier. They are skeletally advanced (not shown in the tables), and they tend to have higher hemoglobins and hematocrits. From the serum and urinary vitamins (ascorbic acid, vitamin A, riboflavin, and thiamine) they do not show evidence of a lower nutrient density, suggesting that they may eat more but not selectively.

LEVEL OF INCOME AND LEVEL OF FATNESS

Having compared the fat and the lean in growth, in size, in development, and in some blood and urinary constituents, let us look next at socioeconomic level and measured fatness. We have data on many thousands of children from *The Ten-State Nutritional Survey* of 1968–1970, and several thousand more from the Preschool Nutrition Survey (courtesy of Dr. George Owen).

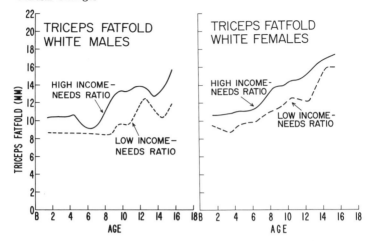

Figure 4. The economic effect on measured fatness in children and adolescents. In both boys (left) and girls (right) the higher income-to-needs ratio (solid line) is associated with greater fatness, and with differences approximating 20 to 25% in measured fatness or calculated as weight of fat (FW).

In general, after the first few years of life and into adolescence, the poor are the leanest, and the more affluent are the fatter (Fig. 4). This generalization is true for girls and for boys (but at different levels of measured fatness), and it is true whether income or parental occupation is the measure.

In brief, boys and girls below the poverty level are the leanest, and boys and girls at median United States income are the fattest. Preschool boys and girls of the lower Warner (occupation/education) ranks (I-II) are leaner than boys and girls of the higher Warner ranks (III-IV).

To complicate the picture of leanness and fatness, there are racial differences in the level of fatness even at the same income levels, with Puerto Ricans in particular exceeding American whites and American negroes or blacks in measured outer fatness. When we look to European fatness data, we find increasingly great discrepancies from our North American fatness percentiles (3).

Not to deflate this part it is still necessary to emphasize that measured fatness differs along income, income/needs, and occupation/education lines. The children of the poor are leaner, the children of the more affluent are fatter, and American boys and girls are (apparently) fatter than their English age-peers.

If the very definition of obesity and leanness is open to some equivocation, let us at least realize that parental income, per capita income, and income relative to needs relate to fatness in childhood and beyond. What we mean by "fat" or "obese" is relative, relative to income, relative to residence, relative in part to race. We may not care to elaborate a grand schema and a single explanation for obesity in the young, knowing that the father's occupation is so much involved.

BODY COMPOSITION OF OBESE AND LEAN CHILDREN

Since obese children are, in general, advanced in both size and development over the average, and the more so as compared with the lean boys and girls, it is scarcely surprising that the obese and the lean differ in the fat-free weight (FFW) as well as in the weight of fat (FW) or in percent fat (%F). Such differences in estimated fat-free weight are shown for white children (of European ancestry) in Fig. 5. Similar fatness-related differences in the FFW separately occur for black boys and girls (of largely African ancestry) and in Mexican-American boys and girls (primarily of Mexican-American ancestry). In terms of the FFW, the obese boys and girls are a year or more ahead of their lean peers.

The values used in Fig. 5 are separately given in Table 5, expressing FFW in kilograms. As seen, the fat-free weight differences tend to increase with increasing chronological age, and at about 10 to 12 years there is a difference of approximately 2 kg (about 7%) between the FFW of the obese and the FFW of the lean.

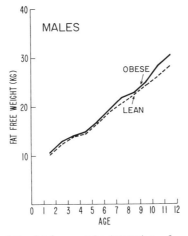

Figure 5. Comparison of the fat-free weight (FFW) in obese boys (heavy line) and lean boys (dashed line). As shown, the obese boys, constituting the upper 15% for triceps fatness for age, have higher fat-free weights than the lean boys (in the lower 15% for triceps fatness). Differences are of the magnitude of 2 kg or 7% at ages 11 and 12.

Table 5   Differences in Body Composition of Obese and Lean Children

Age	Obese N	Median FFW	Lean N	Median FFW	Difference FFW
			Boys		
1	19	9.7	10	9.2	0.5
2	25	11.3	21	11.1	0.2
3	31	14.3	29	13.5	0.8
4	30	13.5	30	14.1	−0.6
5	38	16.2	38	14.8	1.4
6	40	17.7	37	18.1	−0.4
7	46	20.9	45	19.8	1.1
8	41	22.4	45	21.5	0.9
9	43	23.2	38	23.1	0.1
10	46	26.6	45	25.2	1.4
11	44	30.1	39	27.0	3.1
12	37	31.1	39	29.5	1.6
			Girls		
1	21	8.7	15	8.6	0.1
2	25	10.8	23	10.9	−0.1
3	24	11.6	21	12.0	−0.4
4	31	15.0	32	13.2	1.8
5	35	15.7	34	15.7	0.0
6	37	16.5	37	17.2	−0.7
7	40	19.7	38	18.1	1.6
8	39	21.9	38	19.5	2.4
9	41	24.3	40	22.1	2.2
10	40	24.8	41	24.1	0.7
11	37	27.7	37	25.5	2.2
12	34	30.2	36	28.8	1.4

Now not only are the obese boys and girls (at or above the eighty-fifth percentile for triceps fatness) taller than their lean peers, as shown earlier in Fig. 2 and Table 4, but the size of their skeletal components is greater, both with respect to lengths and with respect to radiogrammetrically determined widths. Moreover, computing bone volumes and, from these, estimates of skeletal volume and skeletal weight, obese boys and girls have greater skeletal weights than their lean peers, as shown in Fig. 6. Since the mineral mass, taken as a whole, or with respect to calcium and phosphorous, is proportional to skeletal weight, separate estimates are not given here, and no estimates are made of possible differences in the degree of mineralization of the bone tissue.

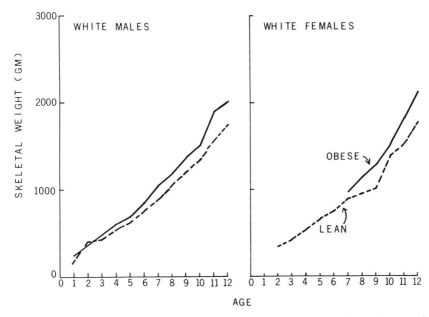

Figure 6. Differences in estimated skeletal weight between obese (heavy line) and lean (dashed line) boys and girls. The obese children are larger, bones are longer, subperiostial diameters are greater, and there is a larger mass of bone in the larger skeletal envelope.

The differences in the skeletal weights (SW) of the obese and lean white boys and girls, depicted in Fig. 6, are paralleled by differences in the skeletal weights of obese and lean American negro (black) boys and girls, but at different levels. This difference is due to the fact that American negro (black) boys and girls are taller than their white age-peers (7) and their (larger) bones have more compact bone, as is also true for American negro adults (2). But within populations of either European or largely African ancestry, the obese children surely have greater skeletal masses and the lean boys and girls have smaller skeletal masses.

Of course at all ages considered the obese children have a far greater percentage of fat (%F), and in the two-component model a smaller percentage of lean (%FFW), since %F plus %FFW of necessity equals 100. So it would be a mistake to argue that the obese have a smaller FFW, as has been done, or that obesity, in childhood or later, is attained at the expense of the lean. The simple fact is that the obese young have a larger fat-free weight and a larger skeletal mass.

Some part of the greater FFW and greater skeletal weight (SW) of obese boys and girls could possibly be a direct consequence of the greater mass they carry, akin to the response to increased g forces shown by experimental animals. Alternatively, the larger FFW and larger SW may simply be a product of the dimensional and developmental advancement associated with hypernutrition. The data simply do not allow us to decide between the two possibilities, though the more parsimonious approach is to favor the second possibility (that is, that the greater FFW is a function of developmental acceleration).

Now there have been attempts to identify two distinct obese types, one associated with a small FFW (small FFW, large FW) and the second associated with a large FFW (large FFW, large FW). Given individual and population differences in FFW, with due correction for the interaction between FFW and FW during the grouping period, it is again difficult to delineate such types other than as the result of chance association. There are obese boys and girls with unusually high fat-free weights (after correction for the FW/FFW correlation during development) and there are obese boys and girls with rather low fat-free weights for their fatness and developmental status, but whether there are two valid biotypes is problematical.

Mostly we can say that obese boys and girls have larger fat-free weights and larger skeletal masses, and that the opposite is true for the lean boys and girls. For the most part these differences between obese and lean appear to be due to the dimensional and developmental differences between them.

POPULATION DIFFERENCES AND LEVELS OF CHILDHOOD FATNESS

Now the labels "obese" and "lean," whether defined in weight terms or in fatness terms, are inevitably specific to a given population, and for the greater part specific to a particular income group. Comparing poor and rich, or Americans and English, we find differing proportions of obese and of lean at different ages (3), and this applies also to populations of different geographical origins (3).

Comparing American white children we have studied (of European derivation) and American negro boys and girls (of largely African ancestry), differences in fatness level, and therefore the proportion that may be termed obese, are apparent throughout. As shown in Fig. 7, black males are fatter from 1 through 4, and then systematically leaner through late adolescence and beyond. The fatness picture is similar for black females in infancy (when they are fatter than the white infants) and through adolescence (when they are leaner). On a population basis, therefore, relative fatness is not systematic from the age of walking to the present age

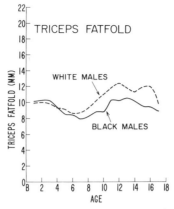

Figure 7. Black-white differences in measured fatness (triceps fat folds) from infancy through adolescence in malese. After age 4, the boys of largely African ancestry (solid line) are systematically leaner, though part of the difference in fatness is related to income or income relative to needs (3).

of voting. So relative fatness need not be programmed early, and then consistent with the early program thereafter.

In the United States, American negroes (or blacks) and American whites have markedly different incomes, even among low-income people. It is therefore appropriate to eliminate the income effect from the comparison by selecting subjects of comparable low incomes, then using the income-to-needs ratio of Orshansky (10), and straddling the officially defined poverty level of 1.0. When this is done, to remove the income effect as much as possible, the differences in fatness shown in Fig. 7 are still most apparent, as in Fig. 8. For thousands of black boys and girls through age 18,

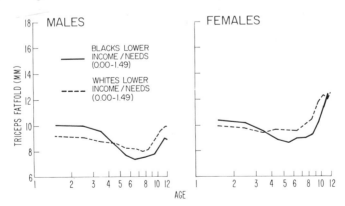

Figure 8. Black-white differences in triceps fatness at constant income-to-needs ratio. At the poverty level black boys and girls are systematically fatter than white boys and girls through age 3, and then systematically leaner into adolescence.

and for thousands of white children through age 18, the blacks (heavy line) are fatter as infants, but systematically leaner as children and into adolescence.

Compared with both blacks and whites, the third census category of Puerto Ricans appears to be systematically fatter even at the same poverty-level grouping (with income-to-needs ratios below 1.49) and approximating the poverty line of 1.0. The Puerto Ricans, of West African and Spanish ancestry, are fatter than either the whites (of European ancestry) or the blacks (with some 70% to 80% of West African genes). The proportion defined as obese by either black or white standards is therefore greater, and the number of the lean is in consequence fewer.

These findings are not included either to confuse or to confound, but they do indicate that the very definition of obesity (and of leanness) includes some problems that merit cerebration. Income level or occupation/education certainly has a bearing on the level of fatness and the prevalence of obesity. For the same level of income, or for income relative to needs, populations certainly differ in fatness levels and the prevalence of infantile and childhood obesity. Group norms for appearance and group attitudes toward eating as well as possible genetic differences in fat storage cannot be left out of consideration.

Table 6   Comparative Fatness of Black and White Boys and Girls at Constant Income[a]

| | Boys | | | | Girls | | | |
| | Black | | White | | Black | | White | |
Age	N	Median Fatness	N	Median Fatness	N	Median Fatness	N	Median Fatness
1	22	10.0	37	9.0	24	9.0	66	10.0
2	20	8.0	53	10.0	27	10.0	40	10.0
3	30	8.0	77	10.0	23	10.0	48	10.0
4	39	9.0	61	9.0	30	7.0	76	9.0
5	36	8.0	97	8.0	41	9.0	78	9.0
6	38	7.0	97	8.0	41	8.0	88	10.0
7	42	7.0	103	8.0	39	9.0	102	10.0
8	31	7.0	105	8.0	42	10.0	95	10.0
9	42	9.0	96	10.0	41	9.0	89	11.0
10	28	8.0	110	10.0	31	11.0	76	12.0
11	37	10.0	101	11.0	36	14.0	87	13.0
12	38	9.0	91	10.0	40	12.0	88	13.0

[a] Income $800 to $1600 per capita. All values refer to triceps fat-fold medians.

IS THE OBESE BOY THE FATHER OF
THE OBESE MAN?

The primary reason for the present state of interest in obesity of the young is the assumption that childhood obesity leads to adult obesity. And if adult obesity leads to increased morbidity and earlier mortality, why not nip obesity in the bud?

Conclusive evidence for the channelization hypothesis is hard to come by, even in the Denver, Fels, and Harvard longitudinal studies, where the necessary radiogrammetric data exist. A next-best resource is in adult follow-up studies of earlier public health examinations, as in the recent analysis of Abraham and associates. They show, using relative weight measures, that relatively underweight boys as of 1923 to 1928 tend to be relatively underweight men as of 1970, while increasing degrees of relative overweight in boys are associated in the same individuals with increasing degrees of relative overweight in adulthood (1). This is a trend that they report; it uses relative weight and not measured fatness, and some underweight boys become overweight men (Table 7). But it scarcely contradicts the assertion that the fat boy is the father of the fat man.

Taking the income-related nature of fatness that we have described earlier, such that the poorest boys are the leanest and the more affluent fatter up through median United States income, the same general trend appears in the adult male data. For males in the third through the seventh and eighth decade, the higher the per capita income (through the $2400 per capita category) or the higher the income-to-needs ratio, through 3.0, the fatter they are.

To the extent that the poor remain poor, and those more affluent remain more affluent, there would appear to be a trend toward lifelong constancy in relative fatness in the male.

Table 7   Relationship between Relative Weight in 1923–1928 and 1961–1963 in 717 Males (1)

Relative Weight in Childhood (1923–1928)[a]	Adult Relative Weight (1961–1963)				
	N	95	95–104	105–119	120–χ
95	223	112	64	38	9
95–104	358	94	119	108	36
105–119	117	12	34	48	23
120–χ	19	0	4	4	12

[a] Age 9–13 years at the time of first examination.

THE INCOME-RELATED REVERSAL OF
RELATIVE FATNESS IN THE FEMALE

As described earlier in this chapter, and in some of our other studies, the level of income and the degree of fatness are related variables during the growing period. This is true in both sexes, and in four racial groupings (comparing lower-income and median-income boys and girls of Mexican, European, African, and Puerto Rican derivation) but at somewhat different race-specific levels of fatness. Within the four-race, two-sex, two-income-level comparisons there are no exceptions, and similar trends may be adduced from other population samplings as well.

Logically, one would assume a similar income-related effect on adult fatness, whether on a simple economic basis (more money, more food), on a habitual basis, or following the assumption of early induction of fat-cell size, if not fat-cell number. And so the data fall for the adult male. From below the poverty level, where the males are leanest, through poverty (and an Orshansky index of 1.0) through above-poverty levels and through median income ($2400 per capita up) more affluent men are fatter men.

But, for the female, the data are not so consistent. More affluent women, at median income, are the leanest, and below-poverty women ($800 per capita and below) are the fattest. And this is no product of small sample size, or of a single racial grouping. For some 20,000 adult women of European, Mexican, African, and Puerto Rican ancestry, the generalization is: the greater the income, the less the fat (Fig. 9).

These data may be differently analyzed to show the proportion of obese women (by any useful standard) at successive economic levels (4). Whether defined as relative weight, percent overweight, or the eighty-fifth percentile for fatness, and regardless of the exact standards used, there is but one generalization. The proportion of obese adult women drops as the income level increases, even though in childhood the relationship is exactly the opposite (Fig. 10).

The evidence for less obesity in the more affluent female is not unique to us. Stunkard found the same trend in his Philadelphia area studies. What is unique here (and so justifies bringing adult fatness data into a symposium on childhood obesity) is the evidence of an income-related reversal in relative fatness, such that the leaner poor girl becomes the fatter impoverished woman.

But if the less affluent female is leaner as a child but fatter as an adult, as the data most clearly show, then is obesity imprinted early, either on the fat cells or upon the psyche? Can estrogens deprogram the fat cells, which is unlikely in view of known effects of estrogens on most sub-

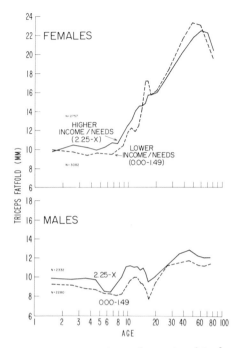

Figure 9. Income-related reversal of relative fatness in white females at adolescence. While the poverty-level male with an income-to-needs ratio of 1.0 is systematically leaner than the median-income male (2.25-χ) at all ages, the lower-income female is considerably leaner before puberty and considerably fatter thereafter. The income-related fatness reversal occurs in black females as well.

cutaneous fat sites? Or are we concerned here with the fashion-dictated concept of sylph and self which affects the poor woman least or even negatively, but causes the more affluent female to haul in her belt, and her fat, as well?

LOWER FAT-FREE WEIGHTS IN OBESE WOMEN

As we have shown, obese boys and girls (being developmentally advanced) tend to have higher fat-free weights and larger skeletal masses during the growing years. Both the total weight of lean (FFW) and the dry skeletal weight or the mineral masses are of higher magnitude in those who represent the upper reaches of fatness for subadult age and sex. But then we find that the adult female is not fat in proportion to her

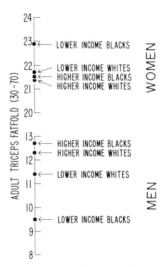

Figure 10. Effects of income on measured triceps fatness in males (below) and females (above). As income increases, males tend toward greater fatness, females to lesser fatness, and black-white differences diminish. The notion of early induction of the level of fatness becomes more questionable if income relates to adult fatness, but in different directions for the two sexes.

juvenile fatness for given income level, but inversely so, such that the leaner socioeconomic groups in childhood yield the fatter females in adulthood (both for blacks and for whites separately). One might then suspect that in the female the magnitude of fat-free weight achieved prior to the end of adolescence would persist thereafter, such that the initially fatter but leaner later girls of medium income would have the higher fat-free weights as adult women.

And so it is with fat-free weight (FFW) as shown in Fig. 11. At all ages considered, the lean women (the lowest percentiles for fatness) tend to have the higher fat-free weights and the obese women (above the eighty-fifth percentile for fatness) tend to have the lower fat-free weights. Taken by themselves, these data might reinforce the notion of a negative relationship between the obese and the lean body mass. Rather, knowing what we do about lifelong trends in fatness, we see these data as further indications that the level of fatness attained early may not persist late, surely for the female and on a lifelong basis for the male. But the fat-free mass and its constituents have greater permanence and some of the differences brought about by association with the degree of fatness may persist, despite the changing nature and magnitude of fatness from earliest life through oldest age.

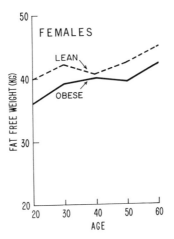

Figure 11. Median fatfree weights (FFW) of obese women (solid line) and lean women (dashed line) derived by subtracting FFW from total body weight on an individual basis. The lower FFW for the obese adult woman is consistent with the income-related reversal of relative fatness in the female (see text and Fig. 9).

DISCUSSION

In our many studies of human growth and development from 1952 to the present, we have not been able to identify a precise upper point in the fatness continuum that automatically spells obesity. And we have been unable to discern a lower point in the fat continuum that automatically designates leanness. While fat and lean children may at times be near-polar extremes in the rate of growth (Δ/yr), in hemoglobin levels and red cell mass, and in serum and urinary vitamins, or in the age at menarche or in epiphyseal union, it is necessary to emphasize the *continuum*. Some of the advantages in size or potential disadvantages of being obese (by the eighty-fifth percentile definition) are shared in part by children of median fatness, at the United States fiftieth percentile. But the median United States child is obese by some other world standards, and at times even our lean are obese by other peoples' percentiles. Our obese infants are relatively lean by the standards of the burgeoning middle class in Salonika or Acapulco.

For adults, we have inherited the 20% overweight definition of obesity from an unknown original source. It has multiple limitations both on an individual basis (ignoring variations in the fat-free weight), and on a group basis (since average adult weight is well above ideal weight). Yet these carpings aside, in adults 20% overweight comes close to the eighty-fifth percentile for fatness. But for infants and for younger children, the 20% overweight rule is either too extreme, or there are far fewer obese infants than there are obese adults. More of the problem is seen in the fact that overweight children are apt to be larger, with larger fat-free weights, and developmentally advanced. So poor is overweight, or relative overweight, or overweight even for size for age, that there is little point in defining childhood obesity except in terms of measured fatness. And even then we hope that the strictures offered in the preceding paragraph will be borne carefully in mind.

Fat children differ from children of median fatness, and those in turn from the statistically lean, in many ways. Fat children tend to be bigger, and within specified limits they have a larger fat-free weight. While we no longer equate bigness exactly with goodness, or at least with bouncing good health, bigness is not necessarily badness either. If we are to restrict fatness, we must accept some consequent restriction in size, a known or probable risk.

Fat boys and girls have higher hemoglobin levels too, a relationship that extends into adulthood and into the later years. Higher hemoglobins and higher hematocrits may not be advantageous, but we should understand this risk as well. If we plan to rethink fatness, we need to rethink the packed red-cell mass as well.

Fat infants and children are not the children of the poor, except in the first few years of life, often with mother-surrogates acting as calorie-pushers to prove their competence and because overfeeding is tranquilizing to feeder and fed. In obese preschoolers and school-age boys and girls, the statistically obese are of middle incomes, and there is a remarkably consistent relationship between parental income (and socioeconomic level) and the degree of fatness of their progeny. If we use median-income families as our reference standard, then the poor have fewer problems of juvenile obesity, but if we employ the impoverished as our reference standard for fatness, obesity and affluence then become identical.

Now it has been suggested (almost to the point of acceptance) that the obese infant is on his inevitable way to becoming an obese adult. But the poor are often fatter in infancy, yet leaner from childhood on. So the fat infant, fat child correlation is but an imperfect one, once we take social class into consideration. The black infant of either sex is the fatter, even at the poverty level, but the black boy and the black girl are leaner than the white boy and the white girl. So the fat infant is not necessarily the antecedent of the fat child.

For males, from age 4 on, those who are more affluent are fatter, at least through median income. This generalization holds at age 5, age 10, age 15, and at age 59, and for whites and blacks and Puerto Ricans and Mexican-Americans.

For females much the same is true, within each genetic population, from nursery-school age through the middle teens. As with male data it is almost as though fatness level were programmed, but at age 4 not age 1. But after the middle teens, higher and lower-income groups of females reverse in fatness—in whites, in blacks, in Puerto Ricans, and (apparently) in Mexican-Americans. The poor are leaner earlier (4 to 15) and fatter later (16 to 80). Those of median income and beyond are fatter earlier and leaner later. How do we program the fat cells to behave like this?

One might invent a hormonal explanation such that testosterone maintains prior fat-cell size but that estrogens reverse the dimensions, making the lean poor girls into fatter poor women, and the fatter more affluent girls into the leaner more affluent adults. Given our exposure to the newspapers, the magazines, and television and the general cult of leanness, it is far more reasonable to suggest that women read the magazines, look at television, and modify their caloric balance accordingly. And so do men, but in the highest income levels.

Now it has been suggested, and argued, and almost accepted that the obese infant is on his or her way to becoming an obese child and, in turn, an obese adult. There is partial confirmation from the Hagerstown, Maryland Survey comparing obesity in preadolescents and their achieved level of fatness into adult life. Confirmatory data from the Harvard (Boston), Denver, Brush Foundation (Cleveland), Berkeley (California), and Fels (southwestern Ohio) longitudinal growth studies at present do not exist. What we do know from cross-sectional studies is more complicated, more confusing, and therefore more like the real nature of things.

So it is difficult to argue from human data that the level of fatness is simply instilled early and that the fatter fat cells then replicate as fat, fat cells. For males beyond infancy such an explanation might seem tenable (though socioeconomic level replicates as well as may cellular fatness). For females, the situation is so reversed that one would have to argue that cellular fatness is reversed by estrogens, so that the fat become lean and the lean become fat.

Under the circumstances, it is premature to assume that adult levels of fatness are instilled early by cells that simply replicate themselves from the baby carriage to the grave. Rather, it is clear that the level of fatness bears a predictable and systematic relationship to the level of income (within an ethnic group) but reverses so paradoxically and impressively in the adolescent female as to boggle all imagination. When the fat become lean and the lean become the fat, on the average, it is even true that (across socioeconomic groups) the fat beget the lean! Under these circumstances we must go back to the real data, redefining our definitions of obesity, further exploring the concomitants of fatness and leanness, recognizing the continuum rather than some point in the Gaussian curve, and ascertaining, from present longitudinal studies and others, that we need to establish exactly what relationships exist, on an individual basis, between the level of fatness in infancy and measured fat (for age, sex, race, and economic level) in adults.

ACKNOWLEDGEMENT

Work described in this chapter was supported in part by contract HSM 21 72 522 with the Center for Disease Control in Atlanta, Georgia, HD 07134 with the National Institutes of Child Health and Human Development, a subcontract with the American Academy of Pediatrics, and a grant from Weight Watchers Incorporated.

We wish to thank Dr. Milton Z. Nichaman and Mr. James Goldsby of the Center for Disease Control for their continued interest, Dr. Charles U. Lowe and the Committee to Advise The Ten-State Nutrition Survey, and Mr. Richard L. Miller of the Center for Human Growth and Development. We also wish to extend thanks to Mrs. Kay Larson for preparation of some of the illustrations, and Miss Dixie L. Farquharson for assistance in manuscript completion.

REFERENCES

1. S. Abraham, G. Collins, and M. Nordsieck, HSMHA Health Rpt. 86: 273 (1971).
2. S. M. Garn, The Earlier Gain and the Later Loss of Cortical Bone. Springfield, Ill.: Thomas, 1970.
3. S. M. Garn, Ecol. Food Nutr. 1: 333 (1972).
4. S. M. Garn, and D. C. Clark, Ecol. Food Nutr. 2: 247 (1973).
5. S. M. Garn, D. C. Clark, and K. E. Guire, Am. J. Phys. Anthrop. 39: in press (1973).
6. S. M. Garn, and J. A. Haskell, Science. 130: 1711 (1959).
7. S. M. Garn, and J. A. Haskell, Am. J. Dis. Child. 99: 746 (1960).
8. S. M. Garn, R. L. Miller, and K. E. Larson in Workshop on Bone Morphometry, A. F. G. Jaworski and E. H. Meema, Eds. Ottawa: 1974.
9. S. M. Garn, and N. J. Smith, J. Pediatr. 83: 346 (1973).
10. M. Orshansky, Soc. Sec. Bull. 28: 3 (1965).
11. F. Quaade, Obese Children. Copenhagen: Danish Science Press, 1955.
12. C. C. Seltzer, and J. Mayer, Clin. Nutr. 38: 101 (1965).
13. The Ten-State Nutrition Survey, 1968-1970. U.S. Dept. of Health, Education, and Welfare Publ. (HSM) 72-8134 (1972).
14. O. H. Wolff, Quart. J. Med. 24: 109 (1955).

3

Modification of Adipose Tissue Fatty Acid Composition

SAMI A. HASHIM, M.D.

Department of Medicine, St. Luke's Hospital Center, and Institute of Human Nutrition, Columbia University, New York, N.Y.

The fat in mammalian adipose tissue is virtually all in the form of triglyceride. The fatty acid composition within the triglycerides consists exclusively of even-numbered long-chain fatty acids in which the chain length varies from 12 to 24 carbon atoms. With the exception of the essential fatty acids (linoleate and those derived from linoleate, such as arachidonate), the mammalian adipose tissue, including that of man, can synthesize fatty acids from nonfat precursors such as glucose and certain amino acids. However, since the human diet usually contains a considerable amount of fat (triglyceride), such a fat may have a profound influence on the fatty acid composition of adipose tissue. This chapter describes how adipose tissue fatty acid composition can be altered by changes in dietary fat.

ADIPOSE TISSUE MOBILIZATION

During the past two decades convincing evidence has been obtained to indicate that adipose tissue releases fat in the form of free fatty acids (FFA) in response to a variety of metabolic, hormonal, and nutritional influences (1-7). An increase in plasma FFA was found during starvation

Supported in part by grant AM-17191 from the National Institutes of Health.

(1,8-10), and in blood draining areas rich in adipose tissue (2). Moreover, plasma glycerol concentration has been found to increase in association with increased levels of plasma FFA, an indication that complete hydrolysis of adipose tissue triglyceride takes place prior to FFA and glycerol mobilization (11-14).

The level of FFA in the plasma appears to reflect in large part the contribution to the body's energy needs from adipose tissue. When the organism is starved, is cold, is stressed, or exercises, more FFA are mobilized from adipose tissue to meet the increased energy demand (2,10,15-17). When the organism eats, there is a rapid fall in FFA concentration reflecting the diminished mobilization of FFA from adipose tissue. In the normal subject, ingestion of carbohydrate is associated with a brisk fall in the plasma FFA concentration, resulting from diminished FFA mobilization from adipose tissue. Thus, under metabolic circumstances favoring deposition, fatty acids are taken up by the adipocytes from circulating chylomicrons (recently ingested fat) and from lipoproteins derived to a major extent from the liver. Since the fatty acids in chylomicrons and lipoproteins are in the form of lipid esters, processing by the adipocytes for entry of fat involves hydrolysis of the ester bonds. Under physiologic conditions of intermittent caloric repletion and fasting, a dynamic state of fatty acid deposition (uptake or synthesis) and mobilization exists in the adipose tissue. Thus, these two processes are determinants of the fatty acid composition of adipose tissue.

DIETARY FATTY ACIDS

The overwhelming proportion of dietary fats consists of naturally occurring triglycerides of which the constituent fatty acids are predominantly long chain. The carbon skeleton of these long-chain fatty acids is even numbered and varies in chain length from 12 to 24 carbon atoms. These fatty acids differ with respect to their chain length, degree of unsaturation, isomerization, and substitution. The edible triglycerides are derived from such sources as land and marine animal tissue, animal milk, bird fats, and fruit flesh and seed fats. The American diet derives 40 to 45% of its caloric content from fat (triglyceride). The fatty acid composition of the usual diet consists principally of oleate (50%), palmitate (20%), stearate (5%), linoleate (15%), longer-chain fatty acids up to C24 including polyenoic acids other than linoleate (7%), and medium and short-chain fatty acids below laurate and down to butyrate (3%). However, the complexity of naturally occurring mixed triglycerides is illustrated by the fact that more than 150 different fatty acids have been isolated from them. Most of these fatty acids occur in small quantities as part of the triglyceride structure.

With the exception of ruminant animals, in general, mammalian adipose tissue fatty acid composition reflects dietary fatty acids. One feature of the ruminant animal is that dietary unsaturated fatty acids can become saturated in the rumen by virtue of bacterial hydrogenation. However, recently it has been possible to enhance the absorption and subsequent appearance of linoleate in the adipose tissue and milk fat of the cow by simply bypassing the rumen.

It has been established that butterfat and coconut oil are endowed with medium and short-chain fatty acids. For example, coconut oil, in which laurate (C12) constitutes approximately 50% of component fatty acids, may contain 10 to 14% medium-chain fatty acids, principally octanoate (C8) and decanoate (C10). Despite their presence in dietary fat and under conditions involving their feeding in triglyceride form as a substantial portion of dietary fat, medium-chain fatty acids (C10, C8, C6, C4) do not appear in adipose tissue. The reason for this is related to their mode of transport after absorption from the intestine.

ROLE OF THE INTESTINE

In recent years significant advances have been made in the basic processes of digestion, absorption, and transport of dietary fats, the long-chain triglycerides (LCT), and the medium-chain triglycerides (MCT). Several excellent reviews and monographs have appeared (18-21). This presentation deals with only certain salient features of the subject in an attempt to emphasize the partitioning role of the intestine in transporting fat after absorption. It is clear that in order for the adipose tissue fatty acids to be modified substantially by dietary fat, the latter must be transported via the chylous route after absorption. In this respect the chain length of the fatty acid determines the intestinal mucosal handling of its transport. Ingested long-chain triglycerides containing fatty acids with a carbon skeleton of 12 carbon atoms or longer are emulsified and transformed by pancreatic lipase to free fatty acids and monoglycerides. The split products are solubilized at the normal intestinal pH into mixed bile acid micelles from which they are absorbed by diffusion. The intestinal mucosa resynthesizes the absorbed fatty acids and monoglycerides into triglycerides. A new process of emulsification begins and a system is elaborated for the transport of the fat out of the mucosa into the lacteals. The products of such a transport system are the chylomicrons, which are particles ranging in diameter from 350 A to 0.5 μ. In this manner, dietary fat reaches the peripheral circulation and from there is transported to a variety of tissues including the adipose tissue.

The transport of ingested medium-chain fat differs strikingly from that of long-chain fats (22-25). In the presence of pancreatic lipase under normal condition, there is extensive intraluminal hydrolysis of MCT, and absorption of this fat seems to occur in the form of FFA. There is evidence that very little, if any, MCT-derived monoglyceride is allowed to remain under the influence of pancreatic lipase. In the absence of pancreatic lipase, the medium-chain fat is present predominantly in triglyceride form in the intestinal lumen and mucosa. However, the exit from the mucosa into the portal venous circulation is mainly in the form of FFA, indicating extensive mucosal hydrolysis of MCT. Thus, unlike the long-chain fatty acids, the absorbed MCT-derived fatty acids do not appear to be esterified to any significant extent in the intestinal mucosa. Rather, they diffuse rapidly into the portal vein as FFA bound to albumin and reach the liver. In the liver, the medium-chain fatty acids are extensively oxidized and do not subsequently appear in significant quantities as FFA or fatty acid ester moieties in the blood leaving the liver (24,26). Thus, animals and humans fed MCT as a major source of fat in the diet display only extremely small quantities of medium-chain fatty acids in their adipose tissue. Figure 1 summarizes in a schematic fashion the chylous and portavenous modes of transport of even-numbered fatty acids following digestion and absorption of LCT and MCT.

MODIFICATION OF ADIPOSE TISSUE IN MAN

It is evident that only dietary fatty acids that are transported into the systemic circulation via the thoracic duct in the form of chylomicron triglycerides are capable of being incorporated into adipose tissue fatty acids. The process of modification of adipose tissue fatty acids in man begins with the first meal. The human infant is born with a certain complement of fat constituted primarily of long-chain fatty acids. The advent of a nontraumatic procedure for sampling adipose tissue in man by needle aspiration (27) and the subsequent analysis of the aspirate by gas-liquid chromatography have allowed for precise determination of adipose tissue fatty acids.

In our laboratory studies were made of the responses of adipose tissue fatty acid patterns to changes in dietary fatty acids in the full-term infant (28). The fatty acid pattern of adipose tissue in a group of 15 infants is shown in Table 1. It is evident that at birth the adipose tissue of infants contains mainly saturated (palmitic C16:0; stearic C18:0; and myristic

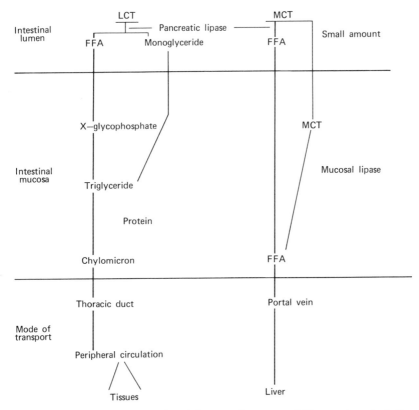

Figure 1. Schema of even-numbered fatty acid transport following intestinal digestion and absorption of long-chain (LCT) and medium-chain (MCT) triglycerides.

Table 1 Fatty Acid Pattern of Adipose Tissue of 15 Full-term Infants at Birth[a]

Fatty Acid	Molar Ratios Percent ± S.D. of Total Fatty Acids
C14:0	3.2 ± 0.2
C14:1	0.5 ± 0.3
C16:0	51.9 ± 3.5
C16:1	9.4 ± 1.1
C18:0	4.1 ± 0.8
C18:1	26.5 ± 1.9
C18:2	0.8 ± 0.7

[a] Fat samples were obtained by needle aspiration of the subcutaneous tissue of the buttocks. The samples were analyzed by gas-liquid chromatography.

C14:0), and monounsaturated (oleic C18:1; and palmitoleic C16:1) fatty acids. Palmitic acid alone was by far the largest component and constituted over 50% of adipose tissue fatty acids of infants at birth. Small amounts, about 1%, of linoleic acid (C18:2) were present.

When a group of six infants were fed a formula diet containing cottonseed oil as the sole source of fat for 3 months, a striking change in the adipose tissue fatty acid pattern occurred (Fig. 2), reflecting the dietary fatty acid input. There was an appreciable incorporation of linoleate reaching 20% at 1 month and up to 39% at 3 months. These changes in linoleate occurred at the expense of the saturated fatty acids palmitate, stearate, and myristate. In contrast, two groups of full-term infants fed either an evaporated milk formula or breast fed had only small to modest rates of incorporation of linoleate. The linoleate contents of samples of the evaporated milk and of breast milk were 0.5 and 8.2% respectively, while those of the adipose tissue of the two groups at three months were 1 and 6% respectively. It is noteworthy that in the group of infants in whom the adipose tissue was enriched substantially with linoleate, there was a transient increase in the demand for the lipid antioxidant α-tocopherol observed after one month on the diet. It is apparent that the rapid incorporation of dietary linoleate in man is seen only when linoleate-rich diets are introduced in the neonatal period.

In the adult human, adipose tissue fatty acid composition generally reflects an overall pattern of long-term intake of dietary long-chain fatty acids. In our laboratory, analysis of adipose tissue aspirates derived from over 100 subjects revealed the following average values in percent of total fatty acids: saturated fatty acids (palmitic, stearic, myristic) 29%; monounsaturated (oleic, palmitoleic) 58%; and polyunsaturated (mainly linoleate) 12%. The most prevalent single fatty acid in adult adipose tissue of Americans consuming the usual American diet is oleic acid (C18:1), comprising approximately 45% of adipose tissue fatty acids. Oleic acid constitutes about 50% of the fatty acids in the American diet. In contrast to the infant, the process of modifying the adipose tissue fatty acids in the adult by diet is indeed slow. When a group of adult subjects from New York City were placed on a diet rich in polyunsaturated fatty acids, particularly linoleate, derived from vegetable oils, the proportion of linoleate in the adipose tissue was doubled (from 11% to 22%) in at least three years (29). Such an incorporation of linoleate occurred at the expense of both saturated and monoenoic fatty acids. Thus, the rate of modifying the adipose tissue fatty acid composition in adult man is extremely slow. Estimates of the halflife of a fatty acid, such as linoleate, in adult humans have ranged up to 750 days (27). In communities outside the United States that consume diets containing different amounts and types of fat,

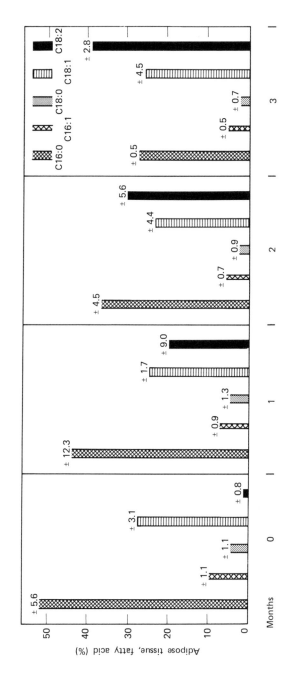

Figure 2. Adipose tissue fatty acids of six full-term infants who received a formula diet containing cottonseed oil (50% linoleate) as the sole source of fat for 3 months. Aspirates of adipose tissue were obtained at birth and at 1, 2, and 3 months.

the adipose tissue fatty acid is suggestive of dietary intake. For example, adults consuming diets extremely low in fat have in their adipose tissue fatty acids that are monoenoic (C16:1; C18:1) as well as saturated fatty acids. On the island of Crete, where the staple fat is olive oil, considerably more oleic acid (62%) and less palmitic acid (15%) was found in the adipose tissue of a group of 200 Cretan men than in American men (30). Thus, in the adult human, adipose tissue can be modified, albeit slowly, by diet.

ENRICHMENT OF DEPOT FAT WITH ODD-CARBON FATTY ACIDS

It is well known that the quantity of carbohydrate in the body is strictly limited to approximately 1 day's supply of energy from liver and muscle glycogen. During periods of starvation, liver glycogen is rapidly depleted and maintenance of glucose homeostasis is dependent on gluconeogenesis from amino acids. Thus, the vast quantity of fat present in the adipose tissue, albeit useful as a source of energy, cannot be converted to glucose. In our laboratory for the first time, it has been possible to store substantial quantities of potentially glucogenic odd-carbon fatty acids.

The first attempt involved the feeding to rats of an odd-carbon medium-chain triglyceride, tripelargonin. Intact rats fed tripelargonin deposited only a small amount (3%) of pelargonate in their adipose tissue. This was not surprising in view of the portal venous transport of pelargonate after absorption from the intestine (22). However, by circumventing the liver and feeding tripelargonin to rats with portacaval anastomoses, it was possible to shunt the transport of pelargonate to the peripheral circulation. In this way appreciable quantities of odd-carbon fatty acids (17%) were deposited in the adipose tissue (31).

An attempt was made to enhance chylous transport of odd-numbered fatty acids by feeding a pure triglyceride of which the fatty acid has been lengthened by one carbon atom over C10. For this purpose triundecanoin (C11:0 triglyceride) was selected (32). Following administration of triundecanoin to thoracic duct cannulated rats, the chyle became lactescent and undecanoate was found in chyle in triglyceride form in quantities accounting for 12% of the administered load. By increasing the proportion of polyenoic LCT in the fat meal, undecanoate transport in chyle triglyceride was enhanced up to 43% of the administered load. Thus it was possible to divert considerable quantities of an odd-carbon fat into the chylomicron transport system.

Enrichment of adipose tissue with striking amounts of odd-carbon fatty acids was achieved in the intact animal by administration of triun-

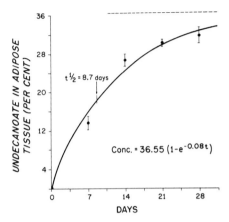

Figure 3. Incorporation of undecanoate (C11) into adipose tissue of rats fed a diet deriving 30% of its calories from fat, a 7:3 mixture of triundecanoin and corn oil, for 4 weeks. Each point represents the mean ± S.E. of six animals. The horizontal interrupted line represents the calculated maximum proportion of undecanoate deposition (37).

decanoin (33-37). Undecanoate enrichment of adipose tissue was rapid in the rat, reaching a plateau in about four weeks (Fig. 3). The fat in the diet of the animals provided 30% of total calories derived from a 7:3 mixture of triundecanoin and corn oil (37). In the dog, also, appreciable quantities of undecanoate appeared in the adipose tissue within four weeks. Moreover, odd-numbered fatty acids longer than C11 appeared, and after 14 weeks the proportion of odd-carbon fatty acids was maintained at 30 to 33%. Following cessation of triundecanoin feeding, the odd-carbon fatty acids were mobilized readily from the adipose tissue into the circulation in the form of FFA. Thus, intestinal transport after absorption for C11 is in the form of chylomicron triglyceride. However, once deposited in peripheral tissues, the mode of transport in the circulation is in the form of free fatty acid (33).

An important aspect of these studies has been the demonstration of the glucogenic potential of the stored odd-carbon fatty acids, presumably by way of the terminal 3 carbon unit, propionate. During prolonged starvation, rats previously fed diets enriched with odd-carbon fatty acids were able to maintain significantly higher levels of liver glycogen and serum glucose than control animals (34,36). If we calculate on the basis of 40% enrichment of adipose tissue with odd-carbon fatty acids, a 260-gm rat would have expanded nonprotein precursors of carbohydrate that would be 8 times the amount of liver glycogen in the same animal. It is emphasized that so far depot fat enrichment with potentially glucogenic odd-carbon fatty acids has been achieved only in experimental animals.

SUMMARY

The adipose tissue is a dynamic organ capable of responding to a variety of metabolic, nutritional, and hormonal influences. The fat within the adipocytes is virtually all triglyceride. Fat leaving the adipose tissue is in the form of free fatty acid, while fat entering the adipose tissue must be in the form of chylomicrons (recently ingested fat) or lipoproteins assembled in the liver. Thus, fatty acid mobilization and deposition in adipose tissue is a dynamic process responding to the energy needs of the organism. It has been shown that adipose tissue fatty acids are predominantly even numbered, varying in chain length from C12 to C24, made up of saturated, monounsaturated, and polyunsaturated fatty acids. In the full-term newborn infant, the saturated fatty acids, particularly palmitate, predominate. Infants receiving formula diets rich in polyunsaturated fatty acids, such as linoleate, rapidly incorporate linoleic acid into their adipose tissue, and within three months the proportion of linoleate in adipose tissue may reach up to 40%. In contrast, American adults starting with 10% linoleate in their adipose tissue and given a linoleate-rich diet incorporate this fatty acid extremely slowly, doubling its concentration in over 3 years. Adults in communities ingesting diets that are low in fat increase their endowment of monoenoic fatty acids in their adipose tissue.

Despite their presence in the diet, in some instances in considerable quantities, the medium-chain fatty acids (below C12) do not appear in the adipose tissue. The reason for this is related to the particular mode of transport by the intestine. After absorption, the medium-chain fatty acids are transported by way of the portal vein and reach the liver where they are extensively oxidized.

In order for a dietary fatty acid to have a chance for deposition in adipose tissue it must be transported via the chyle in the form of chylomicron triglyceride. In recent years, it has been possible to enrich the adipose tissue of animals with appreciable quantities of odd-carbon fatty acids. These fatty acids are potentially glucogenic. Thus adipose tissue enrichment with them would result in a considerable expansion of the non-protein precursors of carbohydrate. The availability of these carbohydrate precursors is important to the animal undergoing starvation, since it will improve the ability to maintain glucose homeostasis. The dictum that "man is what he eats" appears to have a considerable amount of experimental support.

REFERENCES

1. V. P. Dole, *J. Clin. Invest.* **35**: 150 (1956).
2. R. S. Gordon, Jr., and A. Cherkes, *J. Clin. Invest.* **35**: 206 (1956).

3. D. Fredrickson and R. S. Gordon, *Physiol. Rev.* **38**: 585 (1958).
4. E. Wertheimer and E. Shafrir, *Recent Prog. Hormone Res.* **16**: 467 (1960).
5. S. A. Hashim, *Diabetes* **9**: 135 (1960).
6. R. O. Scow, *Handbook of Physiology.* 1965, p. 437.
7. P. Bjontorp, *Adv. Psychosom. Med.* **7**: 116 (1972).
8. S. Laurell, *Scand. J. Clin. Lab. Invest.* **8**: 81 (1956).
9. J. J. Spitzer and H. I. Miller, *Proc. Soc. Exp. Biol. Med.* **92**: 124 (1956).
10. D. W. Walker and N. R. Remley, *Physiol. & Behav.* **5**: 301 (1970).
11. B. Leboeuf, R. B. Flinn, and G. F. Cahill, *Proc. Soc. Exp. Biol. Med.* **102**: 527 (1959).
12. W. S. Lynn, R. M. MacLeod, and R. H. Brown, *J. Biol. Chem.* **235**: 1904 (1960).
13. E. Shafrir, *Bull. Res. Council Israel*, Sect. A: 90 (1960).
14. M. Vaughan, *J. Biol. Chem.* **237**: 3354 (1962).
15. T. B. Van Itallie and A. Khachadurian, *Science* **165**: 811 (1969).
16. P. G. Hanson, R. E. Johnson, and D. S. Zaharto, *Metabolism* **14**: 1037 (1965).
17. M. Mager and P. F. Iampietro, *Metabolism* **15**: 9 (1966).
18. J. R. Senior, *J. Lipid Res.* **5**: 495 (1964).
19. K. J. Isselbacher, *Gastroenterol.* **5**: 78 (1966).
20. A. F. Hofmann, *Gastroenterol.* **5**: 56 (1966).
21. B. Borgstrom, *Proc. Nutr. Soc.* **26**: 34 (1967).
22. S. A. Hashim, K. Krell, P. Mao, and T. B. Van Itallie, *Nature* **207**: 527 (1965).
23. M. R. Playoust and K. J. Isselbacher, *J. Clin. Invest.* **43**: 878 (1964).
24. S. A. Hashim and T. B. Van Itallie, in *Medium Chain Triglycerides*. University of Pennsylvania Press, 1968.
25. S. B. Clark and P. R. Holt, *J. Clin. Invest.* **47**: 612 (1968).
26. R. Scheig, in *Medium Chain Triglycerides*. University of Pennsylvania Press, 1968.
27. J. Hirsch, J. W. Farquhar, E. H. Ahrens Jr., M. L. Peterson, and W. Stoffel, *Am. J. Clin. Nutr.* **8**: 499 (1960).
28. S. A. Hashim and R. H. Asfour, *Am. J. Clin. Nutr* **21**: 7 (1968).
29. G. J. Christakis, S. H. Rinzler, M. Archer, S. A. Hashim, and T. B. Van Itallie, *Am. J. Clin. Nutr.* **16**: 243 (1965).
30. G. J. Christakis, E. L. Severinghaus, Z. Maldonado, F. Kafatos, and S. A. Hashim, *Am. J. Cardiol.* **15**: 320 (1965).
31. R. B. Zurier, R. G. Campbell, S. A. Hashim, and T. B. Van Itallie, *Am. J. Physiol.* **202**: 291 (1967).
32. F. Linares and S. A. Hashim, *Fed. Proc.* **26**: 471 (1967).
33. R. G. Campbell and S. A. Hashim, *Am. J. Physiol.* **217**: 1614 (1969).
34. T. B. Van Itallie and A. K. Khachadurian, *Science* **165**: 811 (1969).
35. M. S. Shin, Ph.D. Thesis, Columbia University, 1969.
36. F. X. Pi-Sunyer, *Diabetes* **20**: 200 (1971).
37. R. G. Campbell and S. A. Hashim, *Proc. Soc. Exp. Biol. Med.* **141**: 652 (1972).

PART 2

Obesity During Critical Periods of Growth

4

Infantile Obesity

WILLIAM B. WEIL, JR., M.D.

Department of Human Development, Michigan State University

Although information about infantile obesity is scarce at present, there is much speculation because of the potential impact that obesity in this age period has on the adult forms of adiposity. In this chapter I discuss four topics: the definition of infantile obesity, its significance, its etiology, and finally its treatment.

First let us define infantile obesity. I have chosen to define infantile by arbitrarily limiting the age group to children under 1 year of age. There is much more difficulty with the term obesity. What we would all like is an absolute measure of body fat in relation to lean body mass; then we could properly quantify the degree of adiposity and make reasonably valid comparisons between various series and experiences. Lacking any usable direct measurement of body fat, we are left with two kinds of problems. The first is to determine an indirect method that can be used to assess body fatness and the other is to determine what degree of fatness we shall choose to call obesity.

The first and most widely used method of defining obesity has been by relating body weight to chronological age. About the only advantage that can be attributed to this method is that both weight and age are easily and inexpensively determined. A mild refinement is to consider weight as it relates to length. This tends to recognize that heavy babies, if long, may in fact have large lean body masses and may not necessarily be obese. Obviously a combination of both length and age adds a little more refinement to the above concept but does not fundamentally change the difficulty inherent in such an approach (13). This difficulty is the inability to distinguish fat from lean body mass when considering total weight.

61

At present the most objective and apparently the best correlated indirect measurement of body fatness is the thickness of the skin folds at specific locations measured with specified equipment. Standards for such measurements as a function of age and weight are now available. If we accept skin-fold or fat-fold thickness as the best measurement available for any wide-scale evaluation, we must still define the degree of adiposity we wish to call obesity.

Going back to weight as the measurement to be considered, Dr. Shukla and others (18) defined individuals as overweight if their relative weight/height for age was 10% greater than the expected standard, and assumed that infants who were 20% over the expected standards were obese. This tended to result in a group labeled as obese that were generally above the ninety-seventh percentile of weight for height at any stated age. Taitz, in a study in Sheffield (19), considered weight-gain rates excessive when they exceeded the ninetieth percentile for children in that area. This is the same standard that Eid used in 1970 (6). Eid also suggested that infants whose weights exceeded the expected by more than 20% should be considered obese. Other authors either have not defined the problem or have separated the obese infant from the overweight infant on the basis of his clinical appearance.

We are left with the problem that, for most babies, height, weight, and chronologic age fall within two standard deviations of the mean, and ordinarily one would not consider such infants overweight or obese. Nevertheless, within this group there are some infants whose lean body mass is relatively small and whose fat tissue is in excess for their lean body mass, while the sum of the two is still within two standard deviations of the average weight for age.

Similarly, infants whose weight exceeds two standard deviations for age are considered to be overweight but may or may not be obese. The infant whose weight is in excess of three standard deviations and whose length is not proportionally increased is much more likely to be obese, but even in such circumstances, without a direct measurement of body fatness or even a good indirect assessment of it, one is probably on shaky ground speaking of such an infant as obese. Dwyer and Mayer in writing on this subject (5) seem to feel that there may be many overweight infants but there are relatively few obese ones. Until we can establish an agreed-upon technique and criteria, we are going to have considerable difficulty speaking intelligently on this subject.

The significance of infantile obesity can be considered from both a short-range and a long-range point of view (20). The short-range problems are debatable, but there are reports that the overweight or obese infant has a greater frequency of illness in general (9) and, perhaps somewhat more clearly, a greater frequency of respiratory illness (21). There is no conclusive evidence that such infants, however, have a higher mortality rate, even though they may have a somewhat increased morbidity rate. More difficult to assess is the question of whether such infants have a greater frequency of psychological problems secondary to their obesity, since psychological problems are considered by most authors to be primary (10) and the obesity often secondary. The reverse hypothesis, however, needs to be considered. The study entitled "Fat Boys Get Burned" is interesting in this regard (22).

The long-range problems are somewhat clearer. The major long-range problem is adult obesity. Several reports indicate that obesity, or at least excessive weight, in infants as young as 6 weeks has a high predictive rate for childhood obesity (6). Another study suggests that 80% of obese children will become obese adults (14). Taken together, the data indicating that obese infants become obese children and that obese children become obese adults, and the concept that an increased number of fat cells develop during infantile obesity (3,4), add up to a fairly gloomy picture of the obese infant's becoming the obese adult with all of the attendant disease processes associated with adult adiposity. The complexities of trying to verify this relationship, however, are well delineated by Abraham and associates (1).

Dr. Stanley Garn has also raised serious questions about the concept that the obese infant becomes the obese child and then the obese adult (8). One of his major arguments involves the "income-related reversal of relative fatness in the female." This refers to the findings in the Ten-State Nutrition Survey, which indicate that poor preadolescent girls are leaner than their not-so-poor counterparts, whereas poor postadolescent women are fatter than the less poor. The problem with data such as that obtained from the Ten-State Survey is that they describe cross-sectional information on large groups of individuals, with the full range of degrees of obesity from very lean to very obese. Let me illustrate how this could be misleading: Although poor young girls are generally leaner than their wealthier peers, there are some moderately obese and very obese girls in the poorer group. These may be the girls who become the most obese poor, adult women. Among the economically more advantaged girls, who as a group are destined to be the leaner adults, the more obese girls may remain obese as adults although the majority of girls that are of a lesser degree of fatness may get leaner as adults and thus lower the higher-income group's mean. What this would suggest is that the variation in the poor group should diminish relatively with age and the variance for the middle-income group should increase with age.

Alternatively, intergroup class mobility may play a role. In such a situation, the lower-economic-level girl who remains thin as an adult has a greater chance of becoming upwardly mobile and appearing in the higher-income group as an adult whereas the higher-income-level girl who becomes obese may be more likely to be downwardly mobile and appear in the poorer group as an adult.

More important, we may not be working with a single population when we consider the truly obese. If, as will be suggested, there are both genetic and environmental factors in obesity, the obese person may not be expected to respond to social and economic factors in the same manner as the rest of the population. In fact, it would be surprising if he or she did.

Thus, although cross-sectional as well as longitudinal studies can illustrate how the general population behaves in regard to relative degrees of adiposity, those who are genetically oriented toward obesity may behave deviantly under many circumstances. It is quite likely, then, that not *all* obese infants become obese children and not *all* obese children become obese adults. Furthermore, not *all* adult obesity begins with infantile obesity. However, it would seem that the process is not a purely random one and our task in the future will be to determine how often infantile obesity leads to adult obesity and how often adult obesity derives from infantile obesity. Then we must learn to identify the obese infants who will become obese adults and concentrate our efforts there.

For the present, not having gained such foresight, let us direct our attention to all obese infants, since many of them may become obese adults. If we can make this assumption, then the primary time for the treatment of much adult obesity and its related disorders is during the first 12 months of our existence. The management of not only obesity but hypertension, cardiovascular disease, diabetes, and their attendant ills may have to begin during the first 1 to 2% of our life span. Thus the significance looms very large for the setting of appropriate growth patterns, particularly in weight, during infancy.

I would like to cite a single case to illustrate what may be a fairly typical example of our problem. A young man of my personal acquaintance has had a marked problem with obesity. He has classically lost 100 pounds and gained 100 pounds several times. He has been a Weight Watchers client and an instructor. Taken from his baby book are the following notes by his mother:

> Under character traits is the heading "Selfish" and the mother wrote "Only with food."
>
> Under "New foods" at 11½ weeks, she wrote "Needed more food to fill uptakes nicely."

At 8 days, she noted "Hungry—eats too eagerly."

At 9 months, "Is an exceptionally good eater and has no dislikes."

At 2 years, "Enjoys eating with a rare enthusiasm in children."

And at 3 years, "Strong love of fattening foods."

Let us now turn to the problem of etiology. If ever there were a multi-factorial problem, infantile obesity is certainly one. The major thesis in our department of human development at Michigan State University is that the individual is the product of his genetic potential and the inter-relationships between this and his internal and external environment, throughout the period from conception to death. This thesis is depicted in Fig. 1. The specific factors, as they relate to the development of obesity, are illustrated in Fig. 2.

As shown on the left of the diagram, the male and female DNA combine to create a unique individual who, if he is to become obese, will do so because he has consumed an excessive number of calories, has less than normal physical activity, has some peculiar abnormal utilization of calories, or has some combination of these three factors. I have placed decreased activity in the middle because I believe this is probably the major functional aspect of the problem we are dealing with.

That there is a genetic factor in obesity seems reasonably clear from the study of children of obese parents who are raised away from their natural parents and those who are raised in their own family setting. No one of these studies is without alternative interpretation but considering

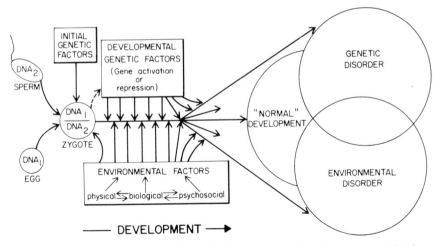

Figure 1. Nature and nurture—relationship between genetic and environmental information during human development.

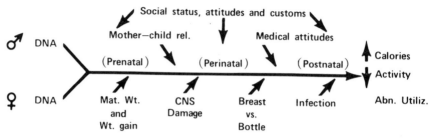

Figure 2.   Etiology of infantile obesity.

them together, one is led to at least suspect some element of genetic influence in the creation of obesity (12). Whether this genetic influence is expressed in terms of caloric intake, activity patterns, or caloric utilization remains unknown.

Turning to the environmental factors, I discuss seven as if they were discrete and independent elements in the etiology of obesity. However, I emphasize particularly the interaction that takes place among these variables. This interaction should always be kept in mind, for these elements are inexorably intertwined.

The first of these factors is maternal weight and maternal weight gain during pregnancy. We are becoming increasingly aware that both maternal weight and maternal weight gain are positively correlated with birth weight in both male and female infants (11,16,17). Although it is not clear whether there is a correlation between birth weight and infantile obesity, the fact that obese parents tend to have obese children leads to a positive correlation between maternal weight and maternal weight gain during pregnancy and obesity in infants (whether it is related through birth weight or some other factor). Let me stress, however, that restriction of maternal weight gain in pregnancy is not recommended, since the deleterious effects of such a course of action would most likely negate any possible effect on the obesity problem.

Another factor that has been related to infantile obesity is central nervous system damage. The role such damage might play in the creation of obesity is not clear. Certainly animal work indicates that one can produce hypothalamic lesions, which result in both increased caloric consumption and decreased activity, producing so-called regulatory obesity. On the other hand, the brain-damaged infant may create increased maternal anxiety and, as we shall see, this in turn has been related to obesity. At the moment, then, this factor is listed but its exact role or significance is uncertain.

The next factor is related to breast versus bottle feeding. There seems to be increasing awareness of the fact that bottle-fed babies are more likely to become obese or at least overweight than breast-fed babies (2,15). The mechanism by which this may happen is unclear, but there are several issues that can be raised although not resolved. First the nutrients in the two milks are different and are present in different combinations in any of the commercially prepared infant milk, cow's milk, and human breast milk. Although the caloric density of the various milks fed to infants is about the same, the differing proportion of calories coming from the various nutrient components could conceivably alter metabolic patterns (7) and potentially play a role in the development of obesity. More important, however, is the ability of the infant to relate more closely his intake of calories to his needs when breast feeding. When the child is bottle fed the mother can measure and thus determine how much the infant will consume, since most small infants can probably be overfed (5).

Another important difference appears to be that breast-fed babies generally seem more active than bottle-fed babies. That there are different arousal levels in the two groups of infants is suggested by the work of Bernal and Richards (2) who had mothers keep diaries describing the activities of their infants. Those diaries showed that breast-fed infants spent less time in bed and received more attention from their mothers. Breast-fed infants cried more and this trend was apparent very early, suggesting that the two groups might have differed practically from birth. This leads to another aspect of the bottle versus breast problem, which is that the psychological direction or set of the mother is going to determine to some extent whether to breast feed or to bottle feed and this psychological set may also determine or be closely related to her attitudes toward nutrition. The early introduction of solid foods could be another part of the problem—particularly in bottle-fed babies. This becomes a problem if, as Dr. Mayer and others have suggested, the infant's satiety mechanism is related to the degree of gastric filling, since any particular volume of high caloric density infant foods will contain a larger number of calories than an equal volume of milk. Unless a relatively large volume of quite high caloric density foods is provided, this probably is not a factor of much signifiance. This factor also seems to be relatively unimportant after 6 months of age.

The next factor is that of infection and although fat babies may have more infections, there is a possibility that the child with more infections may become fat. Although this is the opposite of what we might ordinarily expect, for an occasional infant the repeated infections may not interfere with feeding but may produce decreased activity and, more important, heightened anxiety on the part of the mother. In her need to cope with the problem she may attempt to feed the baby more than it requires since this is one thing she can do to create a "healthy baby."

Turning to the factors listed in the upper part of Fig. 2, I have placed a large variety of specific factors under the major heading of "Social status, attitudes, and customs" to indicate that the social system has an overriding impact on the obesity problem. It affects not only the mother-child relationship but also the physician-mother-child relationship. Before I turn to these two, however, I would like to re-emphasize that these social characteristics affect all other factors as well. The initial step in our reaction, that is, the combining of male and female DNA, is affected by social phenomena, since there is a tendency for obese individuals to choose obese partners for marriage and for the creation of children. This sets the stage for obesity, since infants of two obese parents have a much greater likelihood of becoming obese themselves (12). Maternal weight and maternal weight gain are also affected by social values and social class. From the findings of the Ten-State Nutrition Survey, it would seem that prior to adolescence, weight and family income are positively correlated in both males and females. From adolescence onward this relationship between weight and income remains true for males but reverses itself for females, so that the poorer or lower the socioeconomic status of the adult female the more likely such an individual is to be obese.

In spite of the fact that weight as a criterion for health is disappearing in much of our society, it still persists in many places with regard to infants. The reasons for this remain unknown. The phrase, "my what a healthy fat baby" or "my what a healthy chubby baby" is still heard in supermarkets, on street corners, and in front of proud grandparents. I have yet to hear someone say, "my what a healthy skinny baby" yet that is much more likely to be true, at least in the long run. The social value system also determines maternal attitudes toward breast feeding as well as the way in which a mother interacts with her infant, whether by feeding or by playing.

This brings us to the next specific factor—the mother-child relationship. I am indebted to Dr. Norbert Enzer, a child psychiatrist and the chairman of our Department of Psychiatry for a description of his experiences with the mother-child relationship in the case of obese infants. He believes that the obese child is usually the first born or the first born of a new series of children for a mother, so that the infant is the first in a new mother-child relationship experience. For example, this might be the first child in which the mother has a new set of expectations for her infant; the infant may be the first Rh affected baby, the first premature baby, or the first baby with which the mother has toxemia. Alternatively, this might be the first child that the mother plans to nurse or that the mother plans not to nurse.

Typically, though, the mother does plan to nurse but usually has ambivalent feelings about it. Nursing is often begun under these circumstances but fails in a few weeks, with the rationale that the baby does not seem to be getting enough to eat, that the mother's supply of milk is inadequate, that her breasts are sore, and that the baby is fussy all the time. On further analysis this fussiness is interpreted by the mother as attempting to "get at her." She sees the baby as angry toward her and she is frightened of this anger in the infant. She finds that a bottle can quiet the baby, for whatever reason, and soon interprets all of the needs of the infant as a need for food. If she does not feed the infant, she interprets the baby's cries as being angry and aggressive. Furthermore, she develops guilt over what she interprets as rejection by the infant, and feels guilty also about her rejection of the infant and her failure to be able to breast feed. The interpretation of anger in the infant is often a projection of her own feelings. This projection combined with guilt is worked out by saying, "see how much I love my baby, I'm busy feeding it all the time." The result is a baby that becomes inactive because of overfeeding and soon develops a passive pattern of behavior. This relatively inactive child is then also left with an inability to distinguish his hunger drive from other drives and to ascertain when he is satiated. Experimental work has indicated that later in life such children are unable to ascertain their gastric-filling volumes.

The final environmental factor is the physician's attitude in dealing with the mother and her obese infant. This is an area in which medical frustration is high, understanding is low, satisfaction is minimal, treatment is uncertain, and the result may very well be a negative attitude on the part of the physician toward the mother and such an infant. This can compound the mother-child problem and may also interfere with the likelihood of therapeutic success in the management of the problem. Depending on the physician's own values, he may or may not consider the overweight and passive infant a problem. If the mother and child are of a different social class than the physician, he may fail to recognize the value system under which the mother is operating and hence may fail therapeutically. Furthermore, the relationship between the doctor and his patient may be altered by the social class of the mother from the standpoint of what *she* considers a health problem and what kind of access she has to the health care system. Considering all these factors and their possible interactions, we can appreciate why infantile obesity is such a complex and difficult problem.

Let us now turn to the final subject of our discussion, which is treatment. One point with which most physicians agree is that treatment must begin early. All possible causative factors must be carefully evaluated. Once the individual case has been assessed, the treatment will be determined by the extent of the problem as the physician sees it.

Clearly the physician cannot himself change the social system, its values, its mores, or its customs, nor is he likely to work a major overhaul of the mother-child relationship (although here he can have some impact). He cannot alter the genetic structure of the child nor can he correct the maternal weight or weight gain that occurred during pregnancy or reverse central nervous system damage. If the mother has gone from breast feeding to bottle feeding, he is certainly not likely to get her to go back to breast feeding. If the child is one of the large number who have many infections because of many siblings in the home, the physician may not be able to do much about this either. So what can he do?

The best therapeutic suggestions to date are to adjust caloric intake to the individual infant's needs and to encourage increased nonnutrient stimulation; that is, vocal, visual, and physical stimulation. As pediatricians, we often prescribe feedings on what we consider a rational basis by assuming that a child requires a given number of calories per kilogram of body weight per day; we work out formulas or formula plus solids that will come to this figure. In doing this we may forget the fact that no two babies are alike and that a particular baby will differ from the average either positively or negatively.

If the child in fact requires more food than we have suggested, this soon becomes apparent and the mother is likely to offer it the additional calories. On the other hand, should the infant require fewer calories than we have prescribed, the mother is unlikely to reduce the feedings but is more likely to overfeed the infant and begin the inevitable cycle that often leads to an overweight child and at times to frank obesity. Thus we need to assess each child carefully and perhaps prescribe calories on the low side of the expected amount rather than at the average level. Certainly if obesity is developing, we must examine the caloric intake in terms of weight, linear growth, and the activity pattern that this child demonstrates. If, after examining these aspects of the child, it seems reasonable to reduce the caloric intake, this should be done.

It is difficult to cause an infant to be more active; on the other hand one can certainly encourage the mother to increase her interaction with the infant, to increase the amount of stimulation the infant receives, and to learn to accept as normal infant behavior the child who is awake at times other than when being fed or when hungry.

If one must treat the extremely obese infant, it is probably more effective to do so in a controlled environment such as a hospital. Here the mother can be taught to discriminate the baby's needs, to comfort the infant with activities other than feeding, and in other ways to react appropriately to the infant's drives. The goal is to train the mother rather than to treat her, to demonstrate for her methods of interacting with her child, to help her understand what the child is doing when he cries, and to distinguish the various cries that her infant has. Eventually the feelings that this mother has for her infant may change and she may establish a more positive relationship between herself and her infant in terms of specific activities rather than in terms of fundamental emotional modification. Such intensive programs have been successful in the past and must be considered when the obesity is marked.

In summary, I have first attempted to describe the problem of defining the obese infant. I have made clear, I hope, that obesity in infancy is of great significance to physicians—particularly to pediatricians—but even more to the infant himself. I have discussed a variety of environmental factors that may interact with the basic genetic tendency or predisposition to obesity, resulting in decreased activity, which I feel is dominant in the triad of possible primary etiologies, or increased caloric consumption, or possibly in some abnormality of caloric utilization. The environmental elements include maternal weight and weight gain during pregnancy, central nervous system damage of the infant, the contrast between breast and bottle feeding, the presence of recurring infection, and the broad concept of social status, attitudes, and customs, particularly as exemplified in the mother-child relationship and in the medical attitude toward the problem, the patient, and its mother. Therapeutically, I have attempted to consider the factors in etiology as clues to the appropriate level of treatment and have stressed that to be effective, treatment must be begun early, and if treatment is to begin early, the problem must be recognized early. For only if we become increasingly aware of the potential disorders created by excessive adiposity in the infant will we ever have a major impact on the obesity of the adult and the associated deleterious diseases related to obesity.

REFERENCES

1. S. Abraham, G. Collins, and M. Hordsieck, HSMHA Health Rep. **86**: 273 (1971).
2. J. Bernal and M. P. M. Richards, *The Effects of Bottle and Breast Feeding on Infant Development*, 247-252.
3. C. G. D. Brook, *Lancet*: **2**: 624 (1972).
4. C. G. D. Brook, J. K. Lloyd, and O. H. Wolf, *Br. Med. J.* I: 25 (1972).
5. J. T. Dwyer and J. Mayer, *Overfeeding and Obesity in Infants and Children*, Basel: Karger, 1973, pp. 123–152.

6.   E. E. Eid, *Br. Med. J.* **2**: 74 (1970).

7.   S. J. Fomon, E. E. Ziegler, L. N. Thomas, R. L. Jensen, and L. J. Filer, Jr., *Am. J. Clin. Nutr.* **23**: 1229 (1970).

8.   S. M. Garn, D. C. Clark, and K. E. Guire, in *Childhood Obesity*, M. Winick, Ed. New York: Wiley, 1975.

9.   P. D. Hooper and E. L. Alexander, *Practitioner* **207**: 221 (1971).

10. H. E. Jones, *Practitioner* **208**: 212 (1972).

11. D. Z. Kitay, *J. Reproductive Med.* **7**: 251 (1971).

12. J. Mayer, Some Aspects of the Problem of Regulating Food Intake and Obesity, 255–334.

13. D. S. McLaren and W. W. C. Read, *Lancet* **2**: 146 (1972).

14. I. C. S. Normand, *Practitioner* **209**: 444 (1972).

15. *Nutr. Rev.* **31**: 116 (1973).

16. C. H. Peckham and R. E. Christianson, *Am. J. Obstet. Gynecol.* **111**: 1 (1971).

17. J. Pomerance, *Clin. Pediatr.* **11**: 554 (1972).

18. Shukla, H. A. Forsyth, C. M. Anderson, and S. M. Marwah, *Br. Med. J.* **4**: 507 (1972).

19. L. S. Taitz, *Br. Med. J.* **1**: 315 (1971).

20. The Overweight Child, *Br. Med. J.* **1**: 64 (1970).

21. V. V. Tracey, N. C. De, and J. R. Harper, *Br. Med. J.* **1**: 16 (1971).

22. D. W. Wilmore and B. A. Pruitt, Jr., *Lancet* **2**: 631 (1972).

5

Obesity During Childhood

JEAN MAYER, Ph.D.

School of Public Health, Harvard University, Cambridge, Massachusetts

I should like to begin by introducing some facts about regulation of food intake. To the best of our knowledge, a pound of excess adipose tissue is equivalent roughly to 3500 calories. This is true if we gain an extra pound. If we lose an extra pound, however, the relationship does not hold quite as strictly because when we start losing weight, we lose weight that is more hydrated and the calorie equivalent is, therefore, slightly less than 3500 calories. As the weight reduction continues, the weight loss is more and more pure fat. Thus more than 3500 calories may have to be lost in order to continue to lose at the same rate.

Let us remember this figure (3500 calories) because in terms of excessive weight gain, this figure is essential. If a child systematically eats 100 calories a day more than he expends, which is a very small percentage of the total intake, and we are talking about a very active child who eats 2000 calories a day, there is a 5% increase. In an adult man, 100 calories a day represents only a 3% increase. However this is still 3000 calories a month, or the equivalent of 10 extra pounds a year. In the problems of obesity that we are dealing with, in all but the most extreme cases we are in fact dealing with what must be the result of a very small error in adjustment. Even an extra 5 pounds a year, which over a period of 10 years would still amount to 50 pounds, is no more than 50 calories a day.

What we must remember, therefore, is that underlying the errors in regulation of food intake we are dealing with a very specific, very precise mechanism. Thus in discussing obesity we are really looking not for enormous differences, gigantic personality derangements, vast differences from the normal, but for very small systematic differences. This is a hard concept to accept because I think most of us feel that at any one time we are free to decide whether we want to eat more, whether we want to eat less, whether we want to have an extra dessert which has 250 calories, or not, so that in effect we have an illusion of free will.

The best comparison I can think of is the person who is under hypnosis and who is told under hypnosis that when he wakes up he should go and open the window. He is then awakened and he gives some reason why he wants to open the window—he wants to see the parade that is going by, it is awfully hot, it is awfully cold. He has an immediate rationalization for opening the window—he thinks he is doing it of his own free will but in fact his behavior is determined by the fact that he has been hypnotized into doing it. In many ways the regulation of food intake is similar. One is very precisely geared to within a few calories over a period of sufficient time—a cycle which may in the adult be about 2 weeks, as far as we can determine. Indeed at any time one can modify intake, but regulatory mechanisms take over and make it extremely likely that in the periods that follow the opposite type of behavior will make up for the deviation.

At present an enormous amount of work is being done on the mechanisms regulating food intake. About 100 to 150 laboratories throughout the world, a few of them in this country, are studying mechanisms that were scarcely considered a few years ago. Attempts are being made to characterize and locate glucose receptors sensitive to small modifications in carbohydrate metabolism. Glucose receptors have different roles depending on what part of the hypothalamus they are in. This is only a very small part of the regulatory mechanism. For example, certain fibers that exert control over the entire gastrointestinal tract connect the ventromedial area to the nucleus of the vagus. A particular type of glucose receptor is present in the gastrointestinal tract and in the portal vein. Other types of receptors have been identified in the liver. In the central nervous system we now know that both the thalamus and frontal lobes are involved. We are dealing with a mechanism that we are just beginning to understand and that is probably as precise in its general functioning within a fraction of 1% as any of the regulatory mechanisms dealing with hydration or with electrolyte concentration, or with other systems maintaining body homeostasis. However, the cycle of the corrections is very much slower and therefore gives the illusion that we can do a great deal more about it than we can.

The second point, which has already been made by Dr. Weil, but which I want to emphasize, is that oebsity is not a single phenomenon. Twenty years ago, there was a very simple Freudian explanation for obesity. Everything was explained in terms of personality disturbances. Everyone who was fat was still hankering for his mother's breast instead of having graduated into more adult forms of entertainment. We now know that there are 12 or 15 different forms of obesity. There are a number of different types of hypothalamic and other brain lesions that cause obesity. There are a number of metabolic syndromes involved. One, the obese hypoglycemic syndrome, is characterized by extreme obesity, hypercholesterolemia, and diabetes. There is a primary enzymatic defect in adipose tissue, and we think we have identified the lack of a depressor to the enzyme glycerokinase in the adipose tissue. This, in turn, leads to certain well-characterized biochemical abnormalities in the adipose tissue whereby the entrance of glucose into cells is partially blocked. Secondary changes occur in the morphology and the function of the pancreas. There is hyperplasia of the islets of Langerhans and hypersecretion of insulin. In addition, increased lipogenesis occurs in the liver. Finally anti-insulin properties develop in the ventromedial area of the hypothalamus, which explains the high blood sugar, the high insulin level, and the inability of the satiety mechanism to shut off food intake. Although there is a complex series of steps, we are beginning to get a coherent picture. In animals we are beginning to define the etiology of a number of such syndromes. We may assume from what little is known about control mechanisms in man that the situation is at least as complicated as in the mouse.

As we have seen, an obese person is not simply a thin person with a lot of fat added. Dr. Seltzer and I looked at thousands of obese individuals over the years, particularly children of both sexes, as well as adult women, and the picture is striking. There are certain body types associated with obesity and certain body types that are never associated with obesity. What physical anthropologists call dominant ectomorphs never become obese. In fact, they never even get fat. One of the attributes of ectomorphism is, of course, elongation of the skeleton rather than elasticity in its lateral dimensions. If we look at the ratio of the length to the width of the hand, there is a ratio beyond which we will never find an obese person. Among others things, ectomorphs are characterized by a lack of sufficient adipose tissue to accumulate the fat in the first place.

Be that as it may, we have also found people who have satiety feelings that tend to be very much more abrupt, and people whose activity can go down and whose food intake goes down as activity goes down, which is not true of the dominant mesomorph. Inasmuch as body type is inherited, we may assume that there is a very strong genetic component in human obesity, as indeed there is in all obesities that have been studied in experimental and farm animals. This is borne out by some of the studies we have done in Massachusetts, where we have found that for normal weight parents who have children graduating from high school, 7% of these children are obese by our classifications. If one parent is obese, the proportion is 40% and if both parents are obese, the proportion is 80%. For children who have been adopted at birth, we do not find any correlation with the weight of their adoptive parents. This study was of necessity done on a relatively small scale because records of adoption are confidential in Massachusetts and family data are obtainable only on the basis of personal confidences. A very good study was done in London by Withers (1) on a much larger scale with full access to adoption records. He found much the same results with respect to both inheritance of body types and inheritance of obesity; that is, very strong correlation with biological parents and essentially no correlation with adoptive parents, even if the child was adopted at birth.

Do these results mean that environmental factors are not important? No, but they do indicate that over all, sociological factors, social factors are much less important than familial characteristics in our society. In a community where few people do any physical labor anymore and everyone has at least enough calories, genetic factors have a chance to bloom and the phenotype will express the genotype.

In a society where people have to work hard or there would not be enough food, environmental as well as genetic factors would be much more likely to show up than in our society. Incidentally, there have been contradictory results on the relationship of obesity to social class at various ages. We do find that in our area in Massachusetts we have much the same sort of complex correlations with social class in adults that Dr. Stunkard described for New York (2). That is, for women as one goes down in the socioeconomic scale, the rate of obesity goes up. This is a very complex phenomenon because going down in the socioeconomic scale involves differences in ethnic backgrounds as well as economic and educational backgrounds. But generally speaking we find an inverse correlation in adult women. In men the picture is more complicated because the heavy work in our society is done by men in the lower socioeconomic class so here again we find the curious phenomenon that the thinnest people tend to be at the bottom as well as at the top of the socioeconomic scale and there is a bulge in between. This picture represents the fact that in our society the only people who can exercise are the chairman of the board because he can afford to and the janitor because he has to, and in between the amount of physical activity is, in general, more limited.

As for children, in the communities we studied we did not find a correlation between socioeconomic background and proportion of obesity. However, we did find it at puberty among girls, which leads us to believe that the main effect of socioeconomic background is not on the genesis of obesity but rather has to do with pressure to control weight once there is a threat of obesity. In other words, if you have a lot of money you do something about your weight. But it is our feeling that the factor of having money does not have anything to do with whether one is going to get fat in the first place.

In order to discuss obesity, especially in children, we must examine the effect of activity. I have already noted that in experimental animals we have looked at 10 or 12 different kinds of obesity. In the mouse and some other animals we had already found that besides what we call regulatory and metabolic obesities, there were also types of obesities that were mainly due to pushing the animal beyond the limits of adaptation. When the animal was immobilized, even an animal that was not normally obese could get quite fat. Similarly we have looked at strains of animals that get fat only on very high fat diets, Dr. Atkins notwithstanding. We do not have any strains of animals in the laboratory that get fat because they eat too much carbohydrate, but we do have strains of animals that get very fat only on low-carbohydrate diets and on high-fat diets and we have been interested in the mechanisms of these types of obesity. But as regards activity, the results were very striking. We looked to see if we could find the equivalent in men. We also looked for the equivalents in terms of food habits and the proportion of carbohydrate, fat, and protein, and our results in this regard have been uniformly negative. We have found that obese children and obese adults eat the same proportion of carbohydrate, fat, and protein, and in none of these individuals is the effect of distribution of meals through the day and in different amounts related to activity expenditure. The nature of the diet has no effect. But as regards activity, we were struck very early by the fact that when we looked at the height and weight statistics we were getting in the schools, most of the extra weight gain seemed to take place in the fall and winter. The children did not get fatter during the summer. That led to the conclusion that activity was indeed a factor. Most of the children that we looked at did not eat more than nonobese children; in fact, they ate somewhat less but they were far less active. In our first study we compared 28 thin girls and 28 obese girls very carefully. We paired for such factors as height, weight, grade in school, socioeconomic level, and time of onset of menarche for those that had started menstruating. The obese girls were found to eat between 300 and 400 calories less than the nonobese but there was no great thermodynamic mystery because the time they spent on activity—the time they spent on their feet, not lying down or sitting—was one-third as much as the time spent by the nonobese girls. We then did a very extensive study using motion pictures to follow the children in the course of various types of activity. We compared a number of thin girls with a number of fat girls and found that the amount of time that fat girls spent in motion when exercising was only a very small fraction of the time that thin girls spent in motion when exercising. For example, in playing tennis thin girls were in motion 90% of the time when playing singles and fat girls about 50%. Volley ball showed something of the same order. The greatest difference was in swimming, where we felt that the fat girls would do particularly well because they not only have more buoyancy but in the cold waters of New England they also have more insulation, and yet the amount of time they spent actually swimming, when they felt they were swimming, was only about one-third of the time the thin girls spent swimming.

In order to find out what had come first, decreased activity or overfeeding, we studied 31 infants from 0 to 15 months very carefully. We could not conclude that overfeeding caused inactivity. What we did find was that there was no correlation between weight gains in babies and the amount of food they ate. May I add that it is easy to measure what you put in and by collecting diapers it is also easy to study what comes out. The striking phenomenon is that the fatter babies were quiet, placid babies that had moderate intake, whereas the babies who had highest intake tended to be very thin babies, cried a lot, moved a lot, and became very tense. Some of these babies had intakes of up to twice as much as the intakes of some fat babies who were extremely placid. We concluded that some individuals are born very quiet, inactive, and placid and with moderate intake get fat, and some individuals from the very beginning are very active and do not get particularly fat even with high intakes.

Why do obese children not exercise? We are impressed with the fact that many of those who do not exercise seem to have trouble automatizing their motion. In other words, they exercise in nonrhythmical motions. They do well in archery or shotput, and poorly in anything that requires repeated rhythmical activity. Their activity is facilitated by loud music with a very strong rhythm. Of course, that facilitates everybody's activity, but it has a particularly striking effect on many of these children who will move to the music although they do not move the rest of the time. We have been testing the ability to translate a rhythm into motion of the large muscles and it looks as though this is where there may be a difference between obese and nonobese children. I may add that a society where most children sit and watch TV, where nobody walks, where no rhythmical motions are needed, and where no domestic chores are required is a society where we may expect more obese children.

The second factor of etiological significance is related in terms at least of self-acceleration to the effect of obesity on the fat child. Obesity is an obsession of our society. All we need to do is look at magazines, books, or television. Children who are fat are called "fatty" and made very miserable. We have found from such tests as sentence completion, word association, and picture description, that obese children as compared with nonobese showed much the same sort of psychological profile as children studied by Gordon Allport, for instance, to determine the effects of color discrimination in Mississippi (3). In an impressive study of the effect of prejudice, he showed that black girls exhibited a certain triad of symptoms of obsession with self. Everything reminded them of the fact that they were black. The feeling that their fate was not in their hands, that they had no chance to make their own decisions, and their expectation of rejection, which, of course, was accompanied by actual rejection, are very much the same in obese children. Here again, we find an obsession with self-image. Everything reminds them of fat, and they show very clearly an expectation of rejection that is striking. For example, a picture that shows one girl walking toward a group of other girls is interpreted by 100% of the thin girls as a girl walking toward a group of other girls. However, most obese girls see her as a girl excluded from the group of other girls. This expectation of rejection is very understandable. They are, in fact, rejected from all sorts of social activities and in a study Dr. Canning and I did several years ago we found that they are also rejected when applying to college (4). In our society discrimination is exercised against obese children, particularly obese girls, so that an obese girl has one-third as much chance of getting into the college of her choice, if admissions contain an interview, as a nonobese girl. This obviously tends to make the child more and more isolated, more and more unhappy, and more and more inactive, which may have been the problem in the first place. Now what do we do about it? One could generalize: we must do nutrition education, we must teach people the value of food, proper portion size, and the importance of proper preparation of food and a rational diet. Obviously we ought to do that, but if it is true that the majority of obese children suffer not from increased food intake but from decreased activity, then that is obviously something we ought to do something about also. In fact, there is evidence that some children who are getting obese on a relatively low calorie intake show a decrease in rate of growth in height and weight if we further decrease their calorie intake. So there is every advantage in exercising more. We have, in fact, increased the activity of several hundred obese children in a school system in Newton, and we reported a number of years ago that this was an extremely successful experiment where we were able to reduce about 60% of the children. We exercised them every day for 1 hour and the effect was striking and highly significant. I am sorry to have to report that after 4 years of what appeared to be a great success in nutrition education and exercise with very striking significant differences, the federal money ran out, the local community did not take over the program, and the program was allowed to lapse. We have just completed a survey of the same children as compared to their classmates and their controls and found that the effect that we had instilled and that persisted for 4 years while the program was going on had been completely obliterated in the 3 years that the program had been discontinued. Our conclusion is, yes, we can do something about childhood obesity in large groups, but only if we continue to do it. It seems to have very little permanent value in a society that is geared to prevent any child from moving a muscle unless he absolutely insists upon it.

REFERENCES

1. R. F. J. Withers, *Eugen. Rev.* **56**: 81 (1964).
2. P. B. Goldblatt, N. E. Moore, and A. Stunkard, *J.A.M.A.* **192**: 1039 (1965).
3. G. W. Allport, *The Nature of Prejudice.* Cambridge, Mass.: Addison-Wesley, 1954.
4. H. Canning and J. Mayer, *N. Engl. J. Med.* **275**: 1172 (1966).

6

Juvenile Obesity

FELIX P. HEALD, M.D.

Division of Adolescent Medicine, University of Maryland, School of Medicine, Baltimore, Maryland

In both its etiology and its treatment juvenile obesity differs distinctly from adult obesity. Juvenile obesity, which occurs during the developing phase of life, is distinguished biologically by hyperplasia of the adipose tissue and by the fact that a growing organism responds differently to the same stimuli than an adult organism. In addition, the psychological impact of juvenile obesity may have a lasting effect on the patient's life.

In working with Dr. Brandon Hubbard, a surgeon at the University of Maryland who has performed a large number of ileal-bypass operations for intractable obesity, it was noted that almost without exception the adults who come to ileal-bypass surgery because of intractable obesity developed obesity during childhood. These patients, of course, had hyperplasia of the adipose tissue organ in contrast to patients with adult-onset obesity, who had a more normal complement of cells. In my judgment, hyperplasia of the adipose tissue organ does more to explain the natural history and resistance to treatment of juvenile obesity than anything else we have learned about obesity in the last several decades. Although the factor or factors responsible for hyperplasia of the adipose tissue organ have not yet been determined, hypercalorism will play a central role in these investigations.

In this chapter, we concentrate primarily on the interaction between the obese state or excessive adipose tissue and the biological and psychological events of adolescence. From the clinician's chair, I look at histories of patients whom I have observed over a number of years and point out areas of the physical examination that are unusual as they relate to growth and total development. Finally, I look at some aspects of the treatment of

81

the obese adolescent, particularly in the context of the rapidly growing organism and the interaction between this rapid growth and diet, a therapeutic regime designed to induce catabolism of adipose tissue.

In order to understand more critically the effect of obesity on the teenager, let us review some of the characteristics of adolescence. A velocity curve for height is height per unit of time plotted against age in years. In extrauterine life until about age 11, the velocity of growth in height decreases. Then the rate of growth increases sharply during adolescence. The rapidity of change, whether biological or biologically induced psychological changes, is the keystone in understanding adolescence. Since all of adolescent medicine rests on these particular phenomena, it is essential to understand the magnitude of growth during these years. By the time boys and girls reach adolescence, they have achieved about 80 to 85% of their adult height. Therefore, the increments in height for boys, for example, are less significant than those in body weight. In fact, if one considers weight changes between 10 and 18 years, boys almost double their body mass during adolescence. We must remember, therefore, in discussing obesity that the very nature of the juvenile period dictates a gain in weight. With the overweight child we must consider what kind of weight is being gained, for gain in weight in the obese is usually considered gain in fat.

During this adolescent growth spurt, almost all organs participate in the general increase in size. (The two exceptions are lymphoid tissue in both boys and girls and adipose tissue in the male.) Both boys and girls in early adolescence appear to increase their body fat. About midadolescence, girls normally accelerate the deposition of fat whereas boys, in contrast, may even lose body fat in absolute amounts during the last part of the adolescent growth spurt. Therefore, a sharp, sex-related difference in the amount of adipose tissue present usually occurs during adolescence; and by the end of adolescence the female has about twice as much body fat as the male. Under normal conditions, these changes are probably under hormonal control.

Accompanying these bodily changes are important emotional changes catalyzed by pubescence. One of the major developmental tasks of the adolescent is to adjust to a new body, for this is essentially the problem with which teenagers are faced. During this developmental phase, the secondary sexual organs mature and the final molding of the body into its adult female or male form occurs. Whether the teenager is ready to enter into adulthood or whether or not he has a body he is pleased with, these changes still occur.

In addition to undergoing physical changes, the adolescent will also experience certain psychological challenges. For instance, one very important issue that he must cope with is his identity—that is, his relationships with family and peers, the "who am I" task. Although the concept of identity formation may be familiar to all, for the obese this problem may have very special implications.

Another problem with which the teenager must come to terms is that of sexuality. How does the teenager accommodate the more intense sexual drives engendered by puberty? How do the obese and nonobese teenagers regard their bodies? How they perceive what their bodies look like will influence their responses to their intensified sexual drives and how they handle their sexuality. I submit that for the juvenile obese, particularly the teenage girl, that is an especially difficult and demanding problem. For example, a look at clinics with many obese teenagers will show that it is predominantly girls who seek help for obesity. Along with telling us something about the general developmental aspects of adolescence and about the importance of the body to the female, this also tells us something about our culture. Our current culture places a premium on leanness and a penalty on fatness, particularly in women. Teenage girls easily perceive this expectation and many attempt to comply. Compliance with society's expectation for a slim physical appearance may be unusually difficult for the obese teenage girl. Therefore, it is not surprising that under as yet unidentified conditions, certain obese teenage girls develop a poor body image. This distorted body image persists into adult life and impairs normal psychological functioning.

With this brief review of growth and development as a background, let us now turn to some of the highlights of the clinical history and physical examination of obese patients. I would like to discuss briefly four aspects of the history. The first is the family history. There are two general historical patterns that I have observed in juvenile-onset obesity. One is the child with a strong family history of obesity; that is, either the mother or the father, or both, are obese. One of them may have had juvenile-onset obesity, and a further look into their family trees will reveal that their pedigrees are also littered with obesity. Frequently, obesity in these youngsters is detected in late infancy or early childhood and has persisted throughout childhood. When finally examined, as obese adolescents, they are usually severely overweight.

I have found it very difficult to gather accurate historical material for such youngsters, for example, about early eating patterns. In my judgement, mother-infant interaction and its relationship to feeding may be one of the critical issues in the pathogenesis of juvenile-onset obesity. However, to get this information 10 years later requires much time and unusual skill. This area of investigation, from infancy through childhood, has been strangely neglected in the study of human obesity and only in the past several years has it begun to receive the critical attention it needs. However, Bruch, a number of years ago, clearly demonstrated how food is inappropriately used in some mother-infant interrelationships and results in severe and prolonged obesity (1). A second kind of family, which I see much less commonly, is the obese youngster with no family history of obesity. Both mother and father are lean, as are all of the siblings. When an obese child from a lean family appears in my office, I pay very close attention to his developmental history, for I am almost always able to define a specific event in that child's life in which some psychological upset specifically induced hyperphagia and subsequent obesity. Examples that I have seen are surgical operations, such as tonsillectomies or appendectomies, a broken bone, or some definable, developmental trauma, such as the loss of a father or mother by death, divorce, or desertion. Obviously, this probably happens only when the soil is fertile, when the youngster is susceptible to this kind of injury, and certainly not all people are. However, I have learned to pay attention to this kind of family history. These youngsters not only develop hyperphagia, but it is common to find other associated behavioral difficulties, such as hyperactivity, nightmares, emotional outbursts, withdrawal, and depression. Naturally, the clinical investigation and certainly the treatment of such youngsters are quite different from those of children with a strong familiar or hereditary pattern of obesity. As Dr. Mayer indicated earlier, there has been some effort to document the genetic influence on the development of obesity. At this point, the evidence is somewhat circumstantial; and I think we will be able to untangle and unravel the genetic influence only when there is a clearly identifiable gene that produces metabolic abnormalities generating excessive fatness. When such a relationship has been identified, then the genetics of juvenile obesity can be determined.

One question that often arises is "When does obesity actually begin?" From my observation, the three periods apparently most conducive to the onset of obesity are late infancy–early childhood, around the age of 6 years, and during adolescence. However, just why obesity so frequently develops in one of these three developmental stages is not known.

In taking a clinical history, the issue of food intake or hyperphagia will certainly arise. What do we find and what does it mean? Normally, adolescents eat a good deal of food. Therefore, defining actual hyperphagia in adolescence becomes more difficult than in adult life, where caloric requirements are more stable. In general, studies on this subject suggest that children who are obese in fact eat less than those who are not obese. Many of these studies are based on dietary recall, and the findings are difficult to evaluate and believe since the obese are prone to denial.

For example, if one measures how much obese subjects eat at home by the 24-hour recall method, and then in a hospital setting one serves the subjects the same amount of food they maintain that they ate, all of these obese people, without exception, lose weight (2). Therefore, it appears that obese people consistently tend to underestimate their actual intake. Accurate information on caloric intake in the obese must be based on direct observational data. One study of obese teenagers that directly observed caloric intake did show that they ate less and, as a group, were also less active.

An interesting experiment on obesity was undertaken by Schachter. He gathered some studies from literature on both rats and humans that he felt were fairly reliable and compared them in parallel fashion. He found some reports indicating that obese rats and humans ate slightly more than nonobese. Although the obese humans and rats had fewer meals per day, the amount they ate per meal was greater and they ate more rapidly.

In the first clinical interview with a teenager, I usually get relatively little information about food intake. I know that in order to get truly accurate statements, I must see a teenager two, three, or four times and gain his confidence. One of the things I am most struck by in the clinical interview is under what circumstances these youngsters eat. Do they eat when they're hungry? Ironically, most of their eating is *not* induced by hunger. Instead, I frequently get the response, "I'm just bored." We are perhaps beginning to get an explanation for this behavior in the work of Bruch, who in the late 1950s and early 1960s published data indicating diminished perception of internal bodily sensations such as hunger in the obese (3). There is little evidence from her work in human obesity to suggest that the primary stimulus for eating originates from a sensation of hunger. Therefore, it is not surprising that Schachter observed the striking lack of perception of internal stimuli in regulating food intake (4). As a matter of fact, it appears from their work that many of the cues for eating are external and are learned cues. I think these observations are important, and it will be interesting to see how external stimuli to eating fit into the pathogenesis of juvenile-onset obesity.

I would like to call five aspects of the physical examination to your attention. First, a word about diagnosis. Rarely, in my experience, has difficulty in the diagnosis of obesity arisen as an issue. In the grossly obese youngster, the eye alone can usually make the diagnosis. If a baby or adolescent *looks* fat, he usually *is* fat. Skinfold calipers become important in the transitional stage or intermediate stage between normal amounts of adipose tissue and excessive amounts. Now, what about the effect of obesity on the teenager's height? Earlier this century it was believed that during childhood or adolescence obesity was associated with increased height. At any age these subjects all appear to be taller than the norm.

Therefore, if the obese are taller during adolescence or have accelerated height growth at this time, do they, as a group, also have accelerated maturation? There is only one study that gives a clue to this question. Again, data from Dr. Bruch suggest that the adult height of these obese subjects is less than that of the nonobese (5). Although obese subjects grow more rapidly, their epiphyses close sooner; they have less time to grow. Our adult stature is really a function not only of the rate of growth but of how long we have to grow.

A correlate of accelerated bone growth and maturation is earlier pubescence. English data on the mean menarcheal age suggest that menstruation in the obese girl is generally accelerated by 1 year (6). It seems apparent that the obese youngster has less time in childhood to get ready for the period of adolescence and all of its complex developmental tasks. However, just what effect this contracted childhood has on the developing boy or girl is essentially unknown.

One problem that arises from time to time with obese boys is gynecomastia or excessive breast development. Are these breasts abnormal? Should anything be done about them? Usually gynecomastia in the male is defined by an enlarged areola under which lies an abnormally large amount of breast tissue. In the obese, what one is usually dealing with is a fat breast. For a fat breast, without gynecomastia, in the male the treatment is knowledgeable neglect and attention to the problem of obesity itself.

Another problem that arises in the physical examination of the obese is hypertension. It is not uncommon for obese adolescents to be labeled hypertensive. Adipose tissue has a compressibility factor of about 30%, which causes elevated blood-pressure readings. It has been shown that if one records intraarterial pressure or blood pressure at the forearm, the blood pressure will be normal. So be careful about labeling an obese youngster hypertensive if he has a fat arm, for the arm itself may give a pseudo-elevation of blood pressure. Of course, if there is any question, a direct determination of arterial pressure is indicated because hypertension in the young is a very malignant disease (7).

Three aspects of treatment for the obese adolescent are unique to this age group and therefore deserve special emphasis. First, we must remember that adolescence is basically an anabolic period. Yet the successful treatment of obesity of necessity means catabolism. Ideally, a weight-reduction diet would mobilize calories only from adipose tissue, leaving the remaining organs uninvolved in the catabolic process. Unfortunately, even in adults it is not possible to achieve weight reduction without some loss of lean body mass. This is particularly true during puberty, where a different degree of metabolism may be found depending on the stage of growth of the individual teenager. An actively growing boy on 2500 calories with more than an adequate amount of protein can be in negative nitrogen balance. At 1800 calories with the same amount of nitrogen, he can be further in negative nitrogen balance (8). Another example involves two teenagers. One is a 15-year-old girl, 5 years postmenarcheal and biologically an adult woman. The second is a boy at Stage II, or early in his growth spurt. Both are on 1000 calories; both are eating the same amount of protein. The girl is in positive balance; the boy is in negative balance. What these data suggest is that the teenager, during the period of rapid growth, is unusually sensitive to caloric restriction. Now, what exactly is the effect of caloric restriction on growth? During catabolism, should growth slow down or cease altogether? The only study that supports the hypothesis that growth is curtailed is one published in 1955. In a group of obese youngsters whose diets contained different degrees of caloric deprivation and were losing weight at different speeds, it was demonstrated that if the loss of weight was 1% of the body mass over a unit of time, adequate growth could occur. However, if weight loss exceeded 1% of total body mass per unit of time, there was a marked decrease in growth. This is the dilemma we in pediatrics, and particularly those interested in teenagers, face. That is, we must devise a way of monitoring caloric restriction without repressing growth.

Along with the physical treatment of a prescribed diet, the overweight adolescent must be given special psychological consideration. This stems from the fact that unlike many obese adults who have not gained weight until later in life, the juvenile obese are extremely sensitive about their body image. Stunkard has shown that if a group of obese adults is separated into two groups, one a juvenile-onset group and the other an adult-onset group, a significant portion of adults in the juvenile-onset group will have a poor body image (2). He was able to conclude from his data that poor body image developed not during the childhood phase of their obesity, but during adolescence. This was not surprising to me, since I have felt for some time that adolescence is a particularly important period for formation of body image. It is important for those of us who treat teenagers to screen for poor body image. This is very simply done. One can merely ask the youngsters how they think they look when they look into the mirror. Do they like their bodies? Some obese girls will say, "Yes, I like my body, I like myself, I look pretty," and others will say, "I look like an elephant, I look horrible." My guess is again that this distortion of body image develops in susceptible soil; that is, where such derogatory remarks are made as "Susie, if only you would lose 50 pounds, you'd be so beautiful." Well, by implication, she looks ugly; and if she hears this time and again, she begins to believe it. This is a very important issue, I think, with the adolescent. When it is clear that a poor body image is present, serious consideration should be given to a thorough psychological evaluation. Such an evaluation should focus on poor body image and its effect on general psychological functioning, rather than on obesity.

REFERENCES

1. H. Bruch, *Am. J. Dis. Child.* **59**: 739 (1940).
2. A. Stunkard, *Arch. Gen. Psychiat.* **26**: 391 (1972).
3. H. Bruch, *Eating Disorders.* New York: Basic Books, 1969.
4. S. Schachter, *Am. Psychol.* **26**: 129 (1971).
5. H. Bruch, *Am. J. Dis. Child.* **58**: 457 (1939).
6. O. H. Wolff, *Quart. J. Med.,* New Series **24**: 109 (1955).
7. L. Hahn, *Arch. Dis. Child.* **27**: 43 (1952).
8. F. P. Heald and S. M. Hunt, *J. Pediat.* **66**: 1035 (1965).

PART 3

Early Nutrition and Lipid Metabolism

7

The Diagnosis and Management of Hyperlipidemia in the Pediatric Population

A. K. KHACHADURIAN, M.D.

Division of Endocrine and Metabolic Diseases, The College of Medicine and Dentistry of New Jersey, Rutgers Medical School, Piscataway, New Jersey

The positive correlation between hyperlipidemia and atherosclerosis and the possibility that the fatty streak seen in infancy and early childhood could be a precursor of the atherosclerotic plaque have aroused great interest among pediatricians in the problems of diagnosis and management of hyperlipidemias (1,2).

It is customary to start a discussion of hyperlipidemias by reviewing the major lipid and lipoprotein classes of the plasma and the classification of hyperlipidemias based on plasma lipoprotein phenotypes. Information on this area is now part of every textbook and excellent reviews have appeared in the recent literature (3,4,5,6,7). Therefore, I will take the liberty of discussing the subject of lipoprotein phenotypes and classification through my personal experience, emphasizing the difficulties encountered in their use.

Type I hyperlipoproteinemia is characterized by massive postabsorptive chylomicronemia resulting from the inability of the tissues to hydrolyze the triglyceride-rich particles entering the circulation from the gastrointestinal tract. The classical lipoprotein electrophoretic pattern depict-

Supported by a grant from the Lebanese Council for Scientific Research and United States Public Health Grant 5 M01-RR00199-07.

ing this condition shows a dense band at the origin, indicating that the plasma lipid elevation is limited to the chylomicrons. When chylomicrons as well as very low density lipoproteins (VLDL, prebeta lipoproteins which migrate to a prebeta position) are present, the condition is called type V hyperlipoproteinemia. However, a closer look at the electrophoretic strip of many patients with type I shows the presence of prebeta bands of various intensity (3,8). In other words, the border between type I and type V seems to be hazy, with all gradations of the elevations of the two classes of lipoproteins possible. This phenomenon is far from unexpected since chylomicrons are gradually stripped of their triglyceride content and are converted to smaller and faster moving VLDL. The measurement of plasma postheparin lipolytic activity (PHLA) is used as another criterion for the diagnosis of type I. This activity should be absent or very low to be compatible with type I. In many patients with type V there is also a low activity of the PHLA. Unfortunately, technical difficulties preclude an accurate measurement of the PHLA, which is obtained as the difference between total and hepatic lipase activities of the plasma. It thus appears that the absent or very low activity compatible with the diagnosis of type I cannot be safely distinguished from the low activity of type V (9).

Type IV hyperlipoproteinemia, which is characterized by elevation of the VLDL, is often referred to as endogenous hyperlipidemia, implying an overproduction of these particles. When type I children are placed on a diet that contains minimal amounts of fats and is, therefore, a high-carbohydrate diet, they revert to a type IV pattern (3,9). This has been commonly ascribed to carbohydrate induction resulting from an overproduction of VLDL by the liver. However, it is possible that the accumulation of VLDL is due to the deficiency of the lipoprotein lipase. Evidence for this hypothesis includes the fact that infants placed on fat-free intravenous or oral alimentation do not develop elevation of VLDL and, therefore, are not carbohydrate inducible (10). Moreover, parents of type I patients could have a type IV pattern (3,9), indicating that a moderate deficiency in postheparin lipolytic activity could manifest itself as type IV disorder. Finally, the fact that the lipoprotein pattern of a given patient can revert from a type IV to a type V pattern very frequently and the coexistence of these two types in the same family indicate the lack of a diagnositc specificity for these phenotypes.

Whereas types I, IV, and V represent hypertriglyceridemic states with or without hypercholesterolemia, type II is characterized by hypercholesterolemia with normal or moderately elevated triglycerides, types IIa and IIb, respectively. Unfortunately, the plasma triglyceride values separating type IIa from IIb and even from type IV are ill defined and arbitrary. Values of 150 and 220 mg/100 ml have frequently been used to separate

IIb from IIa and IV from IIb. Since the distribution of plasma triglycerides in the population does not show segregations on either side of these values and since plasma triglycerides in an individual subject even in a steady state fluctuate across these lines of separation, it has to be understood clearly that types IIa and IIb (and less frequently type IV) do not represent necessarily different disease entities but should be used solely to describe a given plasma lipoprotein pattern.

The introduction of the phenotypic classification of the hyperlipoproteinemias by Fredrickson, Levy, Lees, and their associates has had a significant impact on our understanding of the hyperlipidemic states. Unfortunately, most physicians have failed to realize that there is no distinct separation between the six phenotypes described and that the same laboratory findings could be diagnosed as different patterns by different physicians. More seriously, the misconception that a phenotype is diagnostic of a given disorder or pathogenic mechanism is very prevalent. In that sense, the indiscriminate use of the system of classification in spite of the cautionary remarks of their originators and others has led to errors in diagnosis and management of patients.

In this chapter I follow a system of classification shown in Table 1 that I have followed over the past 10 years. Needless to say, it suffers from as many uncertainties as the classification based on plasma lipoprotein phenotypes and should be considered only as a convenient way of grouping patients until advances in our knowledge allow us to evolve a system based on pathogenic mechanisms.

SECONDARY HYPERLIPIDEMIAS

Dietary Hyperlipidemias

Epidemiologic and laboratory studies have clearly established the positive correlation between the dietary content of saturated fats and choles-

Table 1   The Classification of Hyperlipidemias

I.   Secondary hyperlipidemias
   1. Dietary
   2. Secondary to other hereditary or acquired disorders, e.g., diabetes, glycogen storage diseases, hypothyroidism, nephrosis, dysglobulinemias, biliary obstruction.
II. Primary hyperlipidemias
   1. Familial hypercholesterolemias
   2. Hypertriglyceridemic hyperlipidemias
      a. Fat induced
      b. Carbohydrate induced
      c. Combined

terol and plasma cholesterol. Until recently, the fact is that this correlation applies to the pediatric age group as well often has been overlooked. There is a dramatic increase in the plasma cholesterol in the neonatal period and infancy. Thus the mean plasma cholesterol level at birth is approximately 70 mg/100 ml, rising to 155 mg at 1 week of age and to 180 mg/100 ml at 1 year. It has been repeatedly demonstrated that in infants fed a formula containing skim milk or polyunsaturated fats the plasma cholesterol levels are significantly lower than in infants receiving human or cow's milk (11,12).

There are relatively few epidemiologic studies comparing plasma lipids in the pediatric age group in various countries. Our limited studies in Lebanon show that whereas values for cord blood cholesterol (67.8 ± 10.1 S.D.) are similar to those found in the United States, plasma cholesterol in the Lebanese high school students is 132 ± 33 and among university students, 173 ± 35, values that are significantly lower than most reported from western countries (13). At this time, such differences must be ascribed to the differences in the dietary patterns.

It is therefore important to take a dietary history in evaluating the plasma cholesterol of the individual. Children from families whose diets are high in animal fats and eggs may have plasma cholesterol levels that overlap significantly with the values in children heterozygous for familial hypercholesterolemia who are on a prudent diet. In this context, it is important to point out that the term "familial" in describing hypercholesterolemia should be used carefully. Hypercholesterolemia in several members of the same family could be due to common dietary habits or genetic causes.

Hyperlipidemia due to Other Genetic or Acquired Illnesses

Table 1 shows a list of the common disorders that must be ruled out before arriving at the diagnosis of a primary hyperlipidemia. Needless to say, a patient with primary hyperlipidemia may have a disease that alters plasma lipids.

The hyperlipidemia in diabetes mellitus has been the subject of many studies. Pathogenic mechanisms include a decrease in plasma PHLA favoring the accumulation of chylomicrons and probably of VLDL, and an increased synthesis of VLDL, either from free fatty acids or from glucose. The lipoprotein phenotype could be V, IV, or IIb and often varies from day to day in the same individual. Control of diabetes with insulin or weight reduction in the obese diabetic often results in rapid declines in plasma lipid level. A decision on the ratio of carbohydrates to fats in the diet must be based on one's estimate of the magnitude of the two pathogenic mechanisms that are operative. If a decrease in PHLA is considered to be the main factor, a low-fat diet should be tried. If carbohydrate induction is suspected, a low-carbohydrate diet is advised. In either case, the dietary fats should have a high ratio of polyunsaturated fats (P/S ratio) and be poor in cholesterol.

Marked hyperlipidemia is frequently present in glycogen storage diseases. The serum is lactescent and electrophoresis may show a type V or IV pattern. The pathogenesis is not well understood. Combatting the hypoglycemia by frequent feedings results in a decrease but not normalization of plasma lipid levels.

In nephrotic syndrome the plasma cholesterol is markedly elevated. Elevations of chylomicrons, VLDL, and LDL may be present with various degrees of severity.

In hypothyroidism, elevation of the LDL is the most frequent pattern, but elevation of chylomicrons and VLDL may be seen.

Hyperchylomicronemia secondary to pancreatitis must be distinguished from pancreatitis seen in children with hereditary PHLA deficiency. History and examination of other members of the family are often helpful. The presence of diabetes mellitus can further complicate the picture. Omission of dietary fat often results in dramatic drops in plasma lipid levels.

PRIMARY HYPERLIPIDEMIAS

In the pediatric population the two forms of primary hyperlipidemias that have been commonly recognized are the lipoprotein-lipase-deficiency hyperchylomicronemia (type I) and fimilial hypercholesterolemia (type II).

Lipoprotein-Lipase-Deficient Chylomicronemia

Attention is drawn to this condition when the infant develops eruptive xanthomatosis, abdominal colic, fever, hepatomegaly, or lipemia retinalis.

The plasma is lactescent and a creamy layer separates when it is left overnight. The fraction of postheparin lipolytic activity that can be inhibited by protamine is very low or absent. The condition appears to be the expression of the homozygous form of a Mendelian autosomal mutant allele. In the heterozygotes, moderate alterations of plasma lipids (types IIb, IV, or V) and of PHLA can be observed. The incidence of the disorder is not known since only severely affected children have been detected, reported, and included in various reviews. The existence of several genotypes with variable severity of expression cannot be ruled out. A low-fat diet results in rapid clearing of the chylomicronemia and is the accepted mode of therapy. It has been mentioned that some infants can tolerate up to 25% of their calories in the form of fat. The plasma triglycerides should be monitored often to avoid levels that may precipitate pancreatitis. In infants who have very low tolerance to dietary fats, medium-chain triglycerides could be used as a source of calories.

Familial Hypercholesterolemias

In the pediatric age group, familial hypercholesterolemia (FH) is by far the most frequent type of primary or genetic hyperlipidemia. Diagnosis is based on hypercholesterolemia, hyperbetalipoproteinemia, and a mode of transmission consistent with a monogenic Mendelian autosomal pattern. In the absence of a more specific marker, it is not possible to tell how many genotypes are grouped under this entity.

The high incidence of familial hypercholesterolemia in Lebanon has given me a unique opportunity to study this disorder and the following discussion is based primarily on our findings in these patients (13,14,15,16).

The Mode of Inheritance

A study based on 55 children with juvenile xanthomatosis, rapidly progressing atherosclerosis, and marked hypercholesterolemia, from 31 families, is entirely consistent with the hypothesis that these children represent the homozygous state for a disorder that is transmitted by a single autosomal gene. In the following discussion, therefore, I distinguish between homozygotes and heterozygotes.

The homozygotes

In homozygotes, the plasma cholesterol is approximately 4 times the normal, the mean value of the initial measurements being $728 \pm$ S.D. 140 mg/100 ml in our patients. The plasma triglycerides are moderately elevated with a mean of 151 ± 83, which is approximately double the value in the normal sibs. Spontaneous fluctuations in the plasma cholesterol and especially in triglycerides are common. The most frequent lipoprotein pattern is type II, but types IIb, III, and IV can be seen in the same individual during periods of hypertriglyceridemia.

The clinical picture is striking, with the appearance and rapid growth of skin and tendon xanthomas in the first decade. Corneal arcus, xanthelasma, and arthritis that affects single or multiple joints, mimicking rheumatic fever, are other features. The erythrocyte sedimentation rate is persistently elevated in the majority of the patients and plasma fibrinogen is above normal.

Atherosclerosis takes a galloping course. An aortic ejection murmur often appears in the first decade and was present in 87% of our patients. The mean age of death in 11 of our patients was 21 years with a range of 13 to 37. In all cases, death was ascribed to coronary atherosclerosis.

Diets high in polyunsaturated fats and low in cholesterol do not alter significantly the plasma cholesterol, but are used in all patients. Cholestyramine, the bile-chelating resin, did not have a hypocholesterolemic effect, but caused a regression of the size of xanthomas in our patients. Cholestyramine (12–24 g/day) plus nicotinic acid (30–100 mg/kg/day) caused a mean drop of 10% in plasma cholesterol and a significant reduction of the size of xanthomas in half of our patients. In the individual patient, there was no correlation between the effect of therapy on the plasma lipids and on size of xanthomas. The effect of therapy on the atherosclerotic process cannot be assessed at present. One of our patients developed angina one year after an almost complete regression of his xanthomas and while still on therapy. Coronary angiogram showed marked narrowing of his vessels.

The heterozygotes

The criterion commonly used for the diagnosis of the heterozygote is a plasma cholesterol that is higher than the upper 5% cutoff point for the given population. Several studies have shown that measurement of the LDL cholesterol can be a better determinant. The condition can be diagnosed at birth by measurement of the cord blood lipids. Values for total cholesterol of 100 mg/100 ml and for LDL cholesterol of 41 mg/100 ml have been used as cutoff points for diagnosis.

In our experience, a significant overlap exists between the plasma cholesterol of heterozygotes and that of the controls. Thus, in the obligate heterozygotes (parents of homozygotes), the plasma cholesterol ranged between 224 and 486 mg/100 ml. A similar scatter is seen in the pediatric heterozygous population and occasionally it becomes difficult to identify the heterozygous child. In one one family where the father had tendon xanthomas and hypercholesterolemia, we had to label as heterozygotes two children who had plasma cholesterol levels of 180 to 200 mg/100 ml, while two other sibs with plasma cholesterol of 90 to 110 mg/100 ml were classified as normals. These findings indicate that the heterozygous form of FH cannot be ruled out by finding a plasma cholesterol within the normal range for the population. Repeating the test after a high-animal-fat diet, comparing the value to that found in other members of the family, and measurement of the LDL cholesterol may help in deciding. A study of the incidence of atherosclerotic complications in heterozygotes with normal plasma cholesterol would be of utmost interest.

The clinical picture, like the plasma levels, is variable in the heterozygotes. Some live to old age without developing xanthomatosis or stigma of atherosclerosis. Others may have tendon xanthomas and corneal arcus in the second decade and develop clinical atherosclerosis in the third or fourth decade. The reasons for these differences in the expression of the gene, even in the same sibship, are not entirely understood. They cannot all be explained by dietary habits. A polygenic mode of inheritance has been invoked to explain these variations. Our genetic studies in subjects with juvenile xanthomatosis speak against this hypothesis. However, the effect of modifying genes and the possibility that several variants of FH exist cannot be ruled out. Until more is known about the metabolic basis of FH and genetic markers are uncovered, discussions will remain in the realm of speculation.

Diet remains the mainstay of management. Several recent studies have shown that modification of the diet starting at birth can cause significant reductions in plasma cholesterol levels. In our experience, most heterozygous children respond to the prudent diet by a decline in plasma cholesterol of 10 to 20% and many reach and maintain levels between 200 and 250 mg/100 ml. Occasionally values as low as 150 mg/100 ml can be observed in younger children. However, with advancing age, the plasma cholesterol rises and the hypercholesterolemic effect of diet becomes less apparent. Large-scale studies on the long-term effects of diet on the plasma lipid level and on the atherosclerotic processes are urgently needed.

In the child with a strong family history of early atherosclerosis and in whom diet alone does not lower the plasma cholesterol below 300 mg/100 ml, we use one of the bile-chelating resins.

Derangement of the Feedback Inhibition of Cholesterol Synthesis in FH

Studies over the past two decades have shown that hepatic cholesterol synthesis is under a delicate feedback regulatory system and is almost entirely shut off by a high-cholesterol diet. Our studies in six homozygotes have shown that a high-cholesterol diet does not suppress the synthesis of cholesterol from acetate in liver slices obtained from these patients (17). Recently we have found similar results in cultured skin fibroblasts (18,19). Studies from several laboratories had shown that the rate of cholesterol synthesis by fibroblasts is inversely proportional to the concentration of cholesterol in the preincubation medium. We found that when fibroblasts are preincubated for 20 hours in lipid-free medium, there is no difference in rates of incorporation of radioactive acetate into cholesterol between fibroblasts of homozygotes, herterozygotes, and normals. However, in cells that are preincubated in the standard medium which contains 10% calf serum (final cholesterol concentration 3.5 mg/100 ml), fibroblasts from homozygotes synthesize cholesterol at rates that are 10 to 20 times greater than in controls, whereas in the heterozygotes the rates are approximately 3 times the controls. When mevalonate is used as a precursor, the differences between homozygotes and normals are greatly reduced, indicating that the metabolic error in FH lies at a pre-mevalonate step. That these differences are not due to artifact is supported by the fact that these differences persist under a wide range of experimental conditions. Preliminary results indicate that the assay can be useful in the detection of heterozygotes and in distinguishing FH from other types of hyperlipidemias. A study of the regulation of cholesterol synthesis, and especially of the enzyme 3-hydroxy-3-methylglutaryl coenzyme A reductase, may elucidate the ultimate metabolic defect in FH and may allow a more rational approach to the therapy of this disorder.

REFERENCES

1. S. Blumenthal and M. J. Jesse, in M. A. Engle, Ed., *Pediatric Cardiology*. Cardiovascular Clinics **4**: 12. 1972.
2. S. C. Mitchell, *Am. J. Cardiol.* **31**: 539 (1973).
3. D. S. Fredrickson and R. I. Levy, in *The Metabolic Basis of Inherited Disease*, Stanbury, Wyngaarden, and Fredrickson, Eds. New York: McGraw-Hill, 1972.
4. D. S. Fredrickson and J. L. Breslow, *Ann. Rev. Med.* **24**: 315 (1973).
5. R. S. Lees, D. E. Wilson, G. Schonfeld, and S. Gleet, *Prog. Med. Genetics* **9**: 237 (1973).
6. R. I. Levy and B. M. Rifkind, *Am. J. Cardiol.* **31**: 547 (1973).
7. N. B. Myant and J. Slack, *Clinics Endocrinol. Metabol.* **2**: 81, (1973).
8. C. J. Glueck, R. I. Levy, H. I. Glueck, H. R. Gralnick, H. Greten, and D. S. Fredrickson, *Am. J. Med.* **47**: 318 (1969).
9. C. A. Hamly, and A. K. Khachadurian. *Ped. Res.* **7**: 387/159 (1973).
10. A. K. Khachadurian, J. O. Sherman, and F. S. Kawahara, *Ped. Res.* **7**: 389/161 (1973).
11. J. M. Darmady, A. S. Fosbrooke, and J. K. Lloyd, *Br. Med. J.* **17**: 685 (1972).
12. C. J. Glueck, and R. C. Tsang, *Am. J. Clin. Nutr.* **25**: 224 (1972).
13. A. K. Khachadurian. *Leb. Med. J.* **25**: 31. (1972).
14. A. K. Khachadurian, in *Protides of the Biological Fluids*, New York: Pergamon, 1972, p. 315.
15. A. K. Khachadurian and S. M. Uthman, in *Protides of the Biological Fluids*, New York: Pergamon, 1972, p. 323.
16. A. K. Khachadurian and S. M. Uthman, *Nutr. Metabol.* **15**: 132 (1973).
17. A. K. Khachadurian, *Lancet* **2**: 778 (1969).
18. A. K. Khachadurian and F. S. Kawahara, *J. Lab. Clin. Med.* (in press).
19. A. K. Khachadurian, *Leb. Med. J.* (in press).

8

A Pediatric Approach to Atherosclerosis Prevention

CHARLES J. GLUECK, M.D.

University of Cincinnati Medical Center, General Clinical Research Center and Lipid Research Center, Cincinnati, Ohio

RONALD W. FALLAT, M.D.

University of Cincinnati Medical Center, Lipid Research Center, Cincinnati, Ohio

REGINALD TSANG, M.D.

University of Cincinnati Medical Center, Fels Division of Pediatric Research and Newborn Division, Children's Hospital Research Foundation, Cincinnati, Ohio

The fact that the groundwork for atherosclerosis may be laid in childhood has been recognized for some years. In 1965, Riesman called for "possible pediatric responsibility in the prophylaxis of . . . atherosclerosis" (1). Subsequently, germinal attention was focused on the pediatric origin of atherosclerosis by Enos (2), Strong, and McGill (3), McMillan (4), and co-workers. These investigators demonstrated the apparent progression

Supported in part by N. I. H. grant 1-RO1-HE-14597-01 (CJG, RT) and by the General Clinical Research Center Grant (#RR-00068-11), by the Fels Institute for Developmental Research, Yellow Springs, Ohio (R.T.) A portion of this work was done during Dr. Glueck's tenure as an Established Investigator of the American Heart Association, 1971–1976.

from fatty streak to fibrous plaque to full-fledged atheromatous plaque and the substantial increments in these changes in middle to late childhood and again in the second to third decade of life. It was apparent from the early data that many atherosclerotic lesions reached a presumably irreversible stage in the third decade of life (2,5). These studies raised the possibility that an approach to atherosclerosis prevention might well have to start in childhood.

HYPERCHOLESTEROLEMIA IN PEDIATRIC POPULATION STUDIES

Paralleling these autopsy series, several population studies reported the frequent appearance of hypercholesterolemia in children. Serum cholesterol levels were above 200 mg% in 13 to 15% of teenagers in Vermont (6) and Iowa (7) and in 33% of teenagers in Wisconsin (8). Godfrey reported from Australia (9) that 32 of 1292 school children had plasma cholesterol levels over 238 mg%. Duplessis noted that 8.9% of white South African children ages 7 to 11 years and 13.9% of those ages 12 to 15 years, had cholesterol levels greater than 260 mg%, whereas only 1% of various groups of nonwhite children were similarly affected (10). Starr (12) reported that 6 to 7% of school children ages 6 to 14 had serum cholesterol concentrations above 220 mg%. Hence, in a series of population studies in children, using 215 to 230 mg% as an upper limit for normal, a considerable number were found to have modest elevations of cholesterol. These studies, which documented the remarkable frequency of elevated cholesterol in free-living pediatric populations, coincided temporally with the autopsy studies mentioned above (2,5), which suggested that the apparent precursors of the mature atherosclerotic plaque might be detected in childhood. Vlodaver (11) suggested that there was a relationship between "structural findings in coronary arteries of children under 10 years and the reported prevalence of coronary heart disease in the corresponding adult population." Furthermore the plasma lipids have substantial impact on morbidity and mortality in adults.

If the genesis of atherosclerosis is in childhood, identification of a subset of the pediatric population at high risk for atherosclerosis might make possible an approach to primary prevention of cardiovascular disease by reduction of elevated cholesterol or triglyceride levels or both. One approach to primary prevention of cardiovascular disease might then begin by identifying children with elevated levels of cholesterol or triglyceride or both.

DIAGNOSIS

In children the two most common hyperlipidemias are hypercholesterolemia, with a primary elevation of cholesterol and betalipoprotein cholesterol (LDL), and hypertriglyceridemia, with a primary elevation of
triglyceride and very low density lipoprotein cholesterol (VLDL). There
are also a small number of children who have elevations of both cholesterol and triglyceride levels with elevations of both LDL and VLDL.

The diagnosis of hypercholesterolemia in childhood can often be established by analysis of cholesterol or LDL cholesterol or both in cord blood.
The studies of Goldstein and associates have suggested a prevalence of
0.45% for heterozygotes with familial hyperlipidemia at birth (13). This
minimal esitmate of the heterozygote frequency of the familial hyperlipidemias was based only on families in which three-generation vertical
transmission was unequivocally demonstrated. Glueck and co-workers
suggested a frequency of approximately 0.9% for familial hypercholesterolemia at birth in a screening study of cord blood cholesterol in 1800
live births (14). Further analysis of hypercholesterolemic children in this
study revealed that 0.44% (15) had three-generation vertical transmission
of hyperlipidemia, so that a minimal estimate of the heterozygote frequency of the familial hyperlipidemias in the Cincinnati study was
approximately 0.44%. Kwiterovich, in a study of children born to parents
with well-documented familial hypercholesterolemia (16), showed that
50% of them had cord blood hyperbetalipoproteinemia, a distribution
consistent with the autosomal dominant transmission of this disorder.

In contrast to these three studies, Darmady and co-workers in England
have been unable to confirm the utility of cord blood screening in the
diagnosis of hypercholesterolemia (17). However, follow-up studies at
ages 1 and 2 by Glueck (15) and Kwiterovich (16) generally tend to confirm the cord blood evidence. Neonates with hypercholesterolemia and
elevated LDL cholesterol, who are shown at birth to have familial hyperlipidemia by virtue of family screening, can be shown at ages 1 and 2 to
have persistent hypercholesterolemia (assuming that these children have
taken an average cholesterol diet) (15,18,19).

There are not yet any systematized studies that document the prevalence of familial and acquired hypercholesterolemia in school children.
Pediatric population studies that measured cholesterol levels but did not
include family screening have suggested that somewhere from 3 to 10%
of school children have cholesterol levels above an arbitrary upper normal limit of approximately 215 to 230 mg% (6–8, 12).

If one does screen for the presence of elevated cholesterol at birth,
during the school years, or at birth and during the school years, it is

important to distinguish between familial and acquired hypercholesterolemia. The strict diagnosis of familial hypercholesterolemia rests upon the documentation of primary hypercholesterolemia with vertical transmission (three generations from grandparent to parent to child) or the documentation of tendon xanthomas with hyperbetalipoproteinemia (15). Because the diagnosis of hypercholesterolemia in children will necessitate long-term diet and perhaps drug therapy, it is necessary to have at least three measurements, taken sequentially over a 6-week period while the child is eating normally, all demonstrating elevations in cholesterol and LDL cholesterol above normal limits adjusted for age (20). In the diagnosis of hypercholesterolemia in childhood, one must also rule out disorders that can cause secondary hypercholesterolemia, mainly nephrotic syndrome or hyperthyroidism. It is also apparent in school children that excess intake of cholesterol and saturated fatty acids can induce hypercholesterolemia in a child from a normal kindred where no other evidence of hypercholesterolemia can be documented (Table 1).

The diagnosis of hypertriglyceridemia in childhood cannot be made by

Table 1   Dietary Management of Hypercholesterolemia and Hypertriglyceridemia in Children

	Hypercholesterolemia	Hypertriglyceridemia
1.	Rule out disease states that can induce elevations of Cholesterol, Triglyceride.	
2.	Obtain adequate 24-hour dietary recall to provide estimation of total calories, cholesterol, ratio of Polyunsaturates/Saturates.	
3.	Family Screening studies.	
4.	*Diet*	
	Less than 200 mg cholesterol.	— Cholesterol restriction not essential.
	P/S 1.5–2/1.	P/S 1.5–2/1.
	Weight reduction not essential.	*Weight reduction essential.*
		If triglycerides remain elevated after weight reduction, then balanced NIH type IV diet.
5.	*Usual response*	
a.	If cholesterol elevated solely because of exogenous cholesterol intake, *all* children will normalize.	a. With weight reduction to ideal body weight, all children will normalize triglycerides.
b.	If familial hypercholesterolemia, most children ages 1–5 will reduce cholesterol to less than 230 mg%. Children ages 6—, about 33% will normalize on diet; about 66% will retain cholesterol above 230 mg%, LDL above 170.	b. If triglycerides elevated at ideal body weight, 90% of children should further normalize on type IV diet.
c.	Young adults (18–30), average drop in cholesterol about 15%.	c. Young adults (18–30), about 60% will normalize on weight loss and/or type IV diet.

measuring cord blood triglyceride. Studies by Tsang and Glueck have shown that children born of parents with well-documented familial hyperglyceridemia do not have elevated cord blood triglyceride levels (21). In contrast to familial hypercholesterolemia where 50% of the children born to parents with documented type II have hypercholesterolemia (16), approximately 20% of children born to parents with familial hypertriglyceridemia will have elevated triglyceride levels in childhood (22). Although the inheritance of hypertriglyceridemia appears to be autosomal dominant (22), a considerable number of children born to families where one parent and a grandparent have hypertriglyceridemia may have the genotype but not the phenotypic expression in childhood. Hence, in a family where familial hypertriglyceridemia is suspected, but the children have normal blood lipids, periodic screening until adulthood is necessary to rule out the presence of the disorder (22). Again, the most rigorous documentation of the familial disorder should rest upon three-generation vertical transmission or extensive horizontal spread in the siblings of the affected parent and child. Diseases that may cause secondary hypertriglyceridemia should be ruled out (nephrotic syndrome, hypothyroidism, poorly controlled juvenile diabetes). Documentation of hypertriglyceridemia in children depends on demonstrating elevated triglyceride levels in at least three consecutive index samples taken from a fasting specimen (12–14-hour fast).

It is also not uncommon to find elevation of both cholesterol and triglyceride levels in children. Glueck and co-workers have recently completed a study evaluating 94 children born to 33 kindreds where the propositus parent had primary elevations of cholesterol, LDL cholesterol, and triglyceride levels (23). Thirty-seven of these 94 children (39%) had some form of hyperlipoproteinemia with either combined or separate elevations of cholesterol and triglyceride. Some children had hypertriglyceridemia with total and LDL cholesterol levels near but below the ninety-fifth percentile for LDL cholesterol in normals. Because of the substantial variation of plasma triglyceride, VLDL, and cholesterol in these children, the apparent phenotype occasionally was type IV or type IIb, with frequent alternation.

WHICH CHILDREN SHOULD BE SCREENED

Since both familial hypercholesterolemia, familial hypertriglyceridemia, and familial combined hyperlipidemia appear to be transmitted as autosomal dominant traits in many families it is important that complete family screening be done after ascertainment of any adult kindred member with primary hyperlipidemia. It is too early to make any firm recommendations about the scope of screening for hyperlipidemia in children. With relatively unlimited resources one might wish to obtain cord blood cholesterol and follow-up determination of plasma cholesterol and triglyceride levels in the child in late elementary school. Perhaps senior high school would be a good time for screening. An ongoing study of familial hyperlipidemias in neonates, first, third, fifth, seventh, ninth, eleventh, and twelfth-grade students in Cincinnati may provide data on the feasibility of screening at various ages.

An alternative approach might be to ascertain kindreds with early morbid or lethal coronary vascular disease and systematically to analyze serum lipids and lipoproteins in children from these kindreds. Tamir and colleagues studied serum lipids and lipoproteins in 64 men who had myocardial infarction before age 40 (24). Thirty of 85 children born to these fathers were found to have elevated cholesterol levels. Glueck and colleagues (25) recently reported a study of 223 children from 70 families where one parent had a myocardial infarction before age 50. Familial hyperlipoproteinemia was documented in 60 of 70 (85%) of the myocardial infarction kindreds. The predominant lipoprotein phenotypes were types IIa, IIb, and IV in 14, 18, and 28 kindreds, respectively. Familial hyperlipoproteinemia was documented in 69 of 223 (31%) of children from kindreds having parental myocardial infarction, with 34 children having type IIa, 10 type IIb, and 25 type IV hyperlipoproteinemia. The common occurrence of familial hyperlipoproteinemia in progeny of parents who had myocardial infarction before age 50 makes possible early recognition and treatment of elevated cholesterol and triglyceride levels and emphasizes the importance of questions about premature myocardial infarction in the pediatric family history. In the study by Glueck (25), the practicing pediatrician was requested to ask only one extra question during the performance of his usual history and physical exam of a new patient and family: "Did either parent or grandparent of the child ever have morbid or lethal myocardial infarction before age 50?" If the answer was positive, screening of lipids and lipoproteins was suggested.

TREATMENT

In addition to the elevations of cholesterol and triglyceride levels that are either familial or acquired secondary to disease states, there are many American children who appear to have elevated cholesterol levels that are related primarily to an excessive dietary intake of cholesterol. Many studies have been done comparing serum cholesterol levels in American school children with levels in children from other population groups whose general diet is much lower in cholesterol and saturated acids. The average plasma cholesterol level in American children in such studies ranges anywhere from 50 to 100 mg% higher than levels in children from countries eating considerably less cholesterol and much less saturated fatty acids. The "elevated" cholesterol levels in these studies of American children represent a small input of familial disorders and a moderate input of environmental disorders, which are primarily related to the average high intake of cholesterol in the American diet. Because the American pediatric diet is relatively high in cholesterol and saturated fatty acids the definition of normal is very different for American children and children living in South America, underprivileged children in South Africa, or children in developing countries. This difference, coupled with a paucity of large pediatric population studies of plasma lipids and dietary habits, makes it difficult to establish normal levels. The plasma cholesterol level at birth in American children ranges between 40 and 165, with an average of about 60 to 70 mg% (15,16). In studies by Kwiterovich and Glueck the ninety-fifth percentile for LDL cholesterol at birth is 42 mg% (15,16). Cholesterol rises rapidly after birth to the 160 to 170 mg% range by age 1 or 2, and rises only slightly between ages 2 and 20 with average levels in American studies reported somewhere between 160 and 180 mg% (6,8,12). In American children the upper limit for normal serum cholesterol levels probably should be less than 220 to 230 mg% (the ninety-fifth percentile for cholesterol in small studies of normal children). Plasma triglycerides have not yet been well determined in large populations of normal children, but as a general rule plasma triglyceride levels much above 130 to 140 mg% probably deserve more detailed scrutiny. If a child has been identified as having an elevation of cholesterol or triglyceride or both, and if other disease states that could cause these elevations have been ruled out with confidence by direct testing, one then could turn first to a dietary approach to management of hyperlipidemia in children (Table 1).

Dietary Approach to Hyperlipidemia in Children

After ruling out the disease states that could cause hypercholesterolemia in school children and teenagers, the family should be screened for documentation of the familial disorders. In our experience in school-age children there are two to three hypercholesterolemic children without evidence for familial hypercholesterolemia for every one with the familial disorder. A dietary history in most of the children with hypercholesterolemia due to excess dietary cholesterol reveals a daily dietary cholesterol intake of 600 to 1200 mg/day, with an average polyunsaturated/saturated

ratio of about 0.3 or 0.4. As summarized by Schubert, the *average* cholesterol intake in many healthy American children is somewhere between
400 and 600 mg/day, with the polyunsaturate/saturate (P/S) ratio of diet
varying from 0.2 to 0.5. In children found in our studies to have hypercholesterolemia without familial evidence (hypercholesterolemia secondary to high-cholesterol diet) we recommend a prudent low-cholesterol
diet (26) containing approximately 200 mg of cholesterol and a P/S ratio
of 1.5. The cholesterol levels of most children with hypercholesterolemia
secondary to dietary cholesterol excess will, on this low-cholesterol diet,
rapidly return to normal (Table 1).

In children with familial hypercholesterolemia we recommend no specific diet until age 1 and, depending on availability of the family for
follow-up study, perhaps until age 2 (18,20). It is always important to
confirm the presence of hypercholesterolemia at age 1 and age 2 before
instituting any cholesterol-restricted diets in children with familial hypercholesterolemia. At age 1 or 2 we use a modification of the National Institutes of Health type II diet (20,28). This diet contains less than 200 mg of
cholesterol and has a P/S ratio of 1.5/1. In our experience, plasma cholesterol levels in 60 to 80% of children with familial type II (ages 1 to 5)
will be normalized by such a diet. Unfortunately, as children with
familial type II grow older they seem to be less responsive to diet. In the
group aged 6 to 12, in our experience, diet alone normalizes cholesterol
in approximately 40% of children, whereas 60% maintain elevated cholesterol levels (20). In the late teens, children with type II act very much
like adults with type II in that the *average* drop in serum cholesterol on
diet is only about 10 to 15% with 20% of children achieving normal
levels. Dietary intervention in type II is remarkably effective in the young
child (15,18,19) and apparently less effective in the older child and teenager. After a 6-month trial of diet in the older child and teenager, with
plasma cholesterol remaining above 275 mg% and plasma LDL cholesterol remaining above 230 mg%, one might consider adding drug therapy
(cholestyramine resin) to the dietary regimen (20,29).

Hypertriglyceridemia in children is considerably easier to treat with
diet than hypercholesterolemia. Again, after ruling out disease states that
can cause hypertriglyceridemia, and after family studies to look at the
familial nature of the disorder, one turns to a dietary approach for management. First and foremost, it has been our experience that weight
reduction to ideal body weight is the *sine qua non* of therapy for hypertriglyceridemia in children (22) (Table 1). In every child with familial
type IV who has been more than 15% above ideal body weight, weight
reduction has quickly reduced triglycerides to normal (assuming that the
child reaches ideal body weight and sustains his weight at that level). If

triglyceride levels remain elevated at lean body weight, a National Heart Institute type IV diet (a balanced proportion of the calories, 20% as protein, 40% as fat, and 40% as carbohydrates, and moderately rich in polyunsaturates) is effective in maintaining normal triglyceride levels (28). In our experience with 25 children documented to have familial type IV, triglyceride levels in 95% have returned to normal with weight reduction and, if necessary, the type IV diet.

In children with combined elevations of cholesterol and triglyceride and a IIb electrophoretic pattern (23), the response to a low-cholesterol diet is similar to that noted for children with hypercholesterolemia without elevated triglyceride levels. Again, weight reduction in these children, if they are obese, is useful in reducing the triglyceride levels.

It should be emphasized that instituting long-term dietary management in children may have extensive psychological or other societal effects; hence it is incumbent upon the physician to have excellent verification of the diagnosis before instituting any diet. There have been recommendations that the diet pattern of the average American child be substantially changed by reducing cholesterol intake to about 300 mg and reducing saturated fatty acid intake (27). The major effect of these suggested changes for normal children would be to diminish cholesterol intake by 50%, to decrease saturated fatty acid intake from the current intake of about 15 to 18% of calories to 10% or less, and to increase polyunsaturated fat from 3 to 5% of calories to 10 per cent. Practically, this would diminish the intake of products such as butter, cheese, and ice cream, reduce the intake of organ meats, and moderately reduce the intake of meats with high levels of saturated fat.

It is not yet clear that a substantial reduction in dietary cholesterol (with an attendant decrease in plasma cholesterol) in children whose plasma cholesterol level is elevated because of dietary cholesterol intake would reduce the eventual risk of developing heart disease later in life in these otherwise normal children. Long-term population studies directed toward this problem have not yet been done; they would be expensive and, for practical purposes, would require a 40 to 50-year longitudinal period of follow-up to document a reduction in cardiac event rate. Such studies would also involve the use of a control group eating a normal American diet.

Our emphasis has been to identify carefully familial hypercholesterolemia and familial hypertriglyceridemia (in contrast to hypercholesterolemia or hypertriglyceridemia secondary to dietary excesses). This enables us to focus on the 0.3 to 2% (15) (speculative estimate) of American children with elevated cholesterol or triglyceride or both. It is also not yet known whether long-term reduction of cholesterol intake in these children will prevent or ameliorate the atherosclerosis to which they are statistically heir. However, moderate dietary cholesterol restriction, coupled with drug therapy in type II children later in life, enables us to normalize cholesterol levels in most of these children (20).

If one may extrapolate from primate studies, normalization of plasma cholesterol (or triglyceride) in children with familial or acquired hyperlipidemias may limit the formation of irreversible atherosclerotic plaques. It may be more difficult to reverse the course of atherosclerosis in the adult who already has a mature population of fibrotic, calcified atherosclerotic plaques, than to prevent its inception in the child who has only the reversible lesions of fatty streaks and young fibrous plaques.

SPECULATION

Dietary management has a substantial role in the long-term management of familial hypercholesterolemia and hypertriglyceridemia in childhood. Whether the normalization of elevated cholesterol and triglyceride levels in children with inherited and acquired hyperlipidemias will reduce the substantial risk of premature atherosclerosis later in life, is not yet known. There is little evidence to suggest that prudent diets have any deleterious side effects, but a watchful stance must be maintained in this area. We particularly concentrate on the well-defined 0.5 to 1% of American children with familial hypercholesterolemia, who are destined to have clinical premature atherosclerosis as adults. Prudent reduction in dietary cholesterol intake for the other 99% of American children might, however, have a beneficial effect in reducing the pandemic of coronary vascular disease in young adults in this country.

REFERENCES

1. M. Reisman, *J. Pediatr.* **66**: 1 (1965).
2. W. F. Enos, R. H. Holmes, and J. Beyer, *J.A.M.A.* **152**: 1090 (1953).
3. J. P. Strong and H. C. McGill, Jr, *J. Atheroscler. Res.* **9**: 251 (1969).
4. G. C. McMillan, *Am. J. Cardiol.* **31**: 542 (1973).
5. J. J. McNamara, M. A. Malot, J. F. Stremple, and R. T. Cutting, *J.A.M.A.* **216**: 1185 (1971).
6. R. P. Clarke, S. B. Merrow, E. H. Morske, et al., *Am. J. Clin. Nutr.* **23**: 754 (1970).
7. R. E. Hodges and W. A. Krehl, *Am. J. Clin. Nutr.* **17**: 200 (1965).
8. R. Golubjatnikov, T. Paskey, and S. L. Inhorn, *Am. J. Epidem.* **96**: 36 (1972).

9. R. C. Godfrey, N. S. Stemhouse, K. J. Cullen, et al., *Aust. Paediat. J.* 8: 72 (1972).

10. J. P. Duplessis, F. R. Vivier, and D. J. DeLange, *S. A. Med. J.* 41: 1216 (1967).

11. Z. Vlodaver, H. A. Kahn, and H. N. Neufeld, *Circulation* 39: 541 (1969).

12. P. Starr, *Am. J. Clin. Path.* 56: 515 (1971).

13. J. L. Goldstein, J. J. Albers, W. R. Hazzard, H. R. Schrott, E. L. Bierman, and A. S. Motulsky, *J. Clin. Invest.* 52: 128 (1973).

14. C. J. Glueck, F. Heckman, M. Schoenfeld, P. Steiner, and W. Pearce, *Metabolism* 20: 597 (1971).

15. R. C. Tsang, R. W. Fallat, and C. J. Glueck, *Pediatrics* 53: 458 (1974).

16. P. O. Kwiterovich, R. I. Levy, and D. S. Fredrickson, *Lancet* 1: 118 (1973).

17. J. M. Darmady, A. S. Fosbrooke, and J. K. Lloyd, *Br. Med. J.* 2: 685 (1972).

18. C. J. Glueck, R. Tsang, W. Balistreri, and R. Fallat, *Metabolism* 21: 1181 (1972).

19. C. J. Glueck and R. C. Tsang, *Am. J. Clin. Nutr.* 25: 224 (1972).

20. C. J. Glueck, R. Fallat, and R. Tsang, *Pediatrics* 52: 669 (1973).

21. R. Tsang and C. J. Glueck, *Am. J. Dis. Child.* 127: 78 (1974).

22. C. J. Glueck, R. Tsang, R. Fallat, C. R. Buncher, G. Evans, and P. Steiner, *Metabolism* 22: 1287 (1973).

23. C. J. Glueck, R. Fallat, C. R. Buncher, R. Tsang, and P. Steiner, *Metabolism* 22: 1403 (1973).

24. I. Tamir, Y. Bojamower, O. Levtow, et al., *Arch. Dis. Child.* 127: 70 (1974).

25. C. J. Glueck, R. Fallat, R. Tsang, and C. R. Buncher, *Am. J. Dis. Child.* 127: 70 (1974).

26. W. K. Schubert, *Am. J. Cardiol.* 31: 571 (1973).

27. Inter-Society Commission for Heart Disease Resources, *Circulation* 42: A-53, A-95 (1970).

28. D. S. Fredrickson, R. I. Levy, E. Jones, M. Bonell, and N. Ernst, *The Dietary Management of Hyperlipoproteinemia: A Handbook for Physicians.* U.S. Dept. of Health, Education, and Welfare. Public Health Service, Washington,, D.C.. 1970.

29. R. J. West and J. K. Lloyd, *Arch. Dis. Child.* 48: 370 (1973).

9

Atherosclerosis and the Pediatrician

GLENN M. FRIEDMAN, M.D.

Papago Buttes Pediatric Center, Scottsdale, Arizona

Atherosclerosis is the disease process underlying the major cause of morbidity and mortality in the industrialized nations of the world. Atherosclerosis in the human aorta is probably universally present in all populations by 3 years of age and is present somewhat later in the coronary arteries in children in populations where the disease process is prevalent in the adult (1). In the United States, this disease process accounts for approximately 50% of the total mortality. For example, in 1969, approximately 2 million people died from all causes but 1 million died from diseases of the heart and blood vessels, basically from atherosclerosis, and 250,000 or 25% of the deaths were premature (below age 65) (2). To project to the living, if this trend continues then one of every 2 children as well as adults will probably eventually be subject to this single disease process. Not included in these mortality statistics are the millions who have had a "coronary" or "stroke" and whose lives will be foreshortened, their productivity and happiness severely affected.

In the heart the disease process has its beginnings with the development of fixed lesions by the second decade of life in those geographic areas where more of the disease process is seen in the adult. New Orleans, for example, is one of these areas (3). The precursors of the fixed lesions, the fatty streaking of the lining of the coronary arteries, might even be present earlier.

The disease process is thought to develop in the following manner (4). In some genetically susceptible individuals (hyper-responders) serum cholesterol levels increase as early as infancy or early childhood when excessive quantities of cholesterol and saturated fat are ingested. An individual with the unusual genetic metabolic aberration type II hyperbeta-lipoproteinemia does not need the excessive dietary intake to produce elevated serum cholesterol levels. In these individuals abnormally high levels are already present at birth in cord blood. After an unknown but varying period this condition of elevated serum cholesterol may gradually produce occlusion of susceptible arteries, for example, the coronary or cerebral artery, leading to atherosclerosis. This process is accentuated and accelerated by other risk factors, such as hypertension, cigarette smoking, obesity, and lack of physical fitness, and leads finally to heart attack, stroke, aortic aneurism, or gangrene.

RISK FACTORS

Each of these five factors—hypercholesterolemia, hypertension, cigarette smoking, obesity, and sedentary living—is involved with atherosclerosis, and thus its etiology is said to be multifactorial. The relative importance of each of the developing risk factors to the disease process in the pediatric age group is unknown. But it is reasonable to assume that each of these risk factors may begin operating in this pediatric age group (5).

Hypercholesterolemia

In the genetic type II individual elevated levels of low-density choles-terol may be present in the cord blood at birth. It is estimated by Glueck that 1 in 150 to 200 births has elevated cholesterol levels (6), a cogent reason for examining the possibility of screening newborns for this condi-tion. We find that significant numbers of infants, children, and young parents, though asymptomatic, already have higher than desirable cho-lesterol levels. In the otherwise normal potential hyper-responder the cause is dietary. At present little detection and no intervention is occur-ring in the pediatric age group among those with even modest risk.

Hypertension

Hypertension in itself is a potent risk factor and for many years may be completely silent. In the United States it is estimated that 23 million people are hypertensive. Approximately one-half are undetected and only about 15% are under adequate medical management (7). Hypertension probably also has its beginnings in childhood, for this condition or its potential is thought to be hereditary, with the children of hypertensive parents having elevated blood pressures and following similar patterns.

A study by Zinner and associates demonstrates the family blood pressure aggregation, both systolic and diastolic, in standard deviation units (8).

It is thought by Dahl that in the susceptible individual excessive salt consumption early in life may be a hypertension-triggering phenomenon (9). Salt intakes of infants, children, and adults in the United States are high (10) and may be a factor in the development of this condition. Hypertension may accelerate the process of atherogenesis by speeding up the rate of cholesterol infiltration of the artery. In itself, it is a potent contributor to strokes and congestive heart failure. The number of children destined to become essential hypertensives is unknown.

Cigarette Smoking

Cigarette consumption in boys and girls between the ages of 12 and 18 is increasing in the United States (11). This is worrisome in another area, for lung cancer and emphysema are also significantly increasing in the United States. Smoking by parents may also have deleterious effects on children through passive inhalation. Elevated blood pressures and pulses (12) as well as increased respiratory illnesses in children have been noted in homes where the parents smoke (13). It should be noted that nothing is known about future carcinogenic, emphysematous, or cardiovascular disease producing effects of passive smoke inhalation on children. The inception of smoking in the child is related to smoking in the parent (14).

Obesity

Obesity and overweight involve from 10 to 50% of our population and from 10 to 30% of adolescents, according to the Ten-State Nutrition Survey (15). Obesity is a potent risk factor associated with a reduction in life span (16) and with diabetes mellitus, and in heart disease it is associated with sudden death and angina pectoris (17). This says nothing of the anxiety, worry over self-image, and money and energy expended in futile attempts at weight reduction. There is a growing body of evidence suggesting that the roots of this condition are to be found in childhood or perhaps even in infancy.

A study by Brook and colleagues demonstrates that infants who are fat by 1 year of age have an increased chance of remaining fat (18).

Adults who were fat in childhood developed a larger number of fat cells than adults whose obesity developed later. The latter had enlarged fat cells, though a normal number of them (19). This increased number of fat cells is thought to be permanent and may be a potent factor in the continuation of later obesity. The etiology of the abnormal positive energy balance producing caloric retention may be either inactivity or excessive caloric intake, possibly relating to faulty eating or sedentary living patterns.

Sedentary Living

It has been said that since 1920 caloric intake in the United States has not been increasing (it has even decreased slightly) but our energy expenditure is gradually being seriously restricted through our technology (Fig. 1). According to the National Adult Physical Fitness Survey conducted in 1972, 45% of American adults do not engage in physical activity for exercise (49 of the 109 million adults) (20). Relatively little is known nationally of physical fitness in our children or adults.

Physical fitness may afford protection against the cardiovascular disease process by opening coronary collateral supply, increasing the caliber of coronary arteries, helping to reduce tension, decreasing triglycerides, decreasing blood coagulability, increasing cardiac efficiency, helping to lower blood pressure, and maintaining a desirable weight (21).

It is estimated that the average child spends several hours watching television. Not only is he probably learning little, but he is being robbed of physical activity. More important, sedentary ways of living are being established. The use of motor bikes and school buses also results in reduced activity in this pediatric age group.

What will happen to the infant in the United States? If present trends continue, there is a 50% or greater chance of his developing an increased serum cholesterol level. There is a greater than 30% chance that he will smoke, a 10 to 20% chance of his being hypertensive, a 20 to 50% chance of his being obese, and perhaps a 45% chance that he will become sedentary (Fig. 2). All of these are associated with a better than 50% chance that he will eventually develop a coronary, or stroke, and this says nothing about other environmentally associated diseases such as lung cancer or emphysema.

- 45% OF AMERICAN ADULTS – NO EXERCISE
- WALKING – MOST COMMON EXERCISE
- BOWLING – MOST COMMON PARTICIPATORY SPORT
- 64% OF ADULTS HAD NO ELEMENTARY SCHOOL PHYSICAL EDUCATION
- ONLY 1 OUT OF 5 ADULTS TOLD BY THEIR PHYSICIAN TO EXERCISE

*FROM NATIONAL ADULT PHYSICAL FITNESS SURVEY 1972**

Figure 1.   Our sedentary living. From National Adult Physical Fitness Survey 1972.

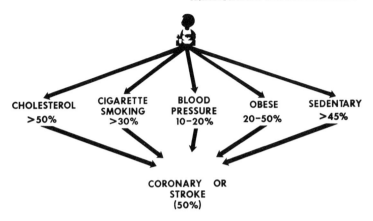

Figure 2.

The implications, interrelationships, and importance of elevated serum cholesterol levels, hypertension, cigarette smoking, obesity, and sedentary living in the pediatric age group are not known (Fig. 3). But since these factors probably are harmful and definitely are not advantageous, and since each has been related to our cardiovascular epidemic as well as other disease processes, it would seem reasonable to proceed to reduce or prevent these factors from developing in the child and the parents without producing anxiety or decreasing the joy of living.

In the face of this massive epidemic destined to involve half or more of our population, a major pediatric priority must be to define those children as well as those parents who are at even modest risk and to help them reduce this risk, first through education, then through personal involvement, finally producing behavioral change. But perhaps more important, we must develop methods of preventing the formation of these risk factors in the first place. It is reasonable to assume that if the child goes through life with low cholesterol levels, does not smoke, is not hypertensive, is not fat, and is physically fit, the chances should be good that he will not have a coronary or a stroke at least in young adult life.

Then why begin lifetime prevention with the child? There are several good reasons:

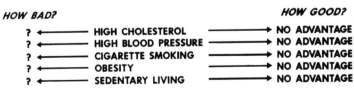

Figure 3.   Cardiovascular risk factors in the child.

● ASSOCIATED "RISK FACTORS" BEGIN IN THIS AGE PERIOD —
  (PATTERNS OF LIVING ARE ESTABLISHED IN CHILDHOOD)

● ATHEROSCLEROSIS DEVELOPS IN THE CHILD.

● ATHEROSCLEROSIS MAY BE MORE "REVERSIBLE" IN THE YOUNG.

● REDUCE "RISK FACTORS" IN THE CHILD ⟶ REDUCE
  "RISK FACTORS" IN THE PARENT.

Figure 4.   Why I start atherosclerosis prevention with the child.

1. The risk factors associated with the development of the disease begin here. Patterns of living are established in childhood.

2. The disease process itself, atherosclerosis, develops in the pediatric age group.

3. Atherosclerosis may be more reversible in the young age group.

4. By reducing developing risk factors in the child, risk factors in the parents probably will also be reduced (Fig. 4).

The family lives together, eats together, exercises together, and perhaps even smokes together. Thus what is needed is a primary prevention program developed for the entire family and not singling out one particular high-risk family member, for risk factors in the children correlate well with those in the parent (8,11,22,23).

SCREENING PROGRAMS IN ARIZONA

In Arizona there are two cardiovascular screening and intervention programs operating at present (Fig. 5). One is in our private pediatric practice and the other is a community program developed by the nutrition section of the State Department of Health.

Our Private Practice Screening Program

Our private pediatric approach, which began in September 1970, now involves more than 3400 middle-class, mainly Caucasian families in Scottsdale, Arizona. It is an ongoing longitudinal study in association with Dr. Stanley Goldberg of the department of pediatrics, University of Arizona College of Medicine. Figure 6 shows the factors that we attempt to measure twice yearly.

Risk factors screened for children include total serum cholesterol levels, blood pressures, subcutaneous fat measurements, maximal endurance tests on the bicycle ergometer, information about the type of milk feed-

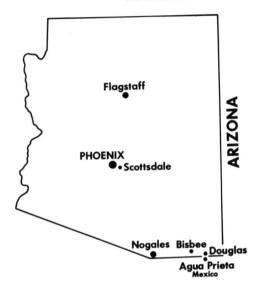

Figure 5.

ing, and exercise history. Parental risk factors screened include total serum cholesterols, blood pressures, subcutaneous fat measurements, exercise history, smoking history, and family history of premature cardiovascular disease and hypertension.

These tests are taken during both well-child visits and minor illness visits. The first is taken when the infant is 1 month old. The parents are given the results of all tests in the hope of increasing their interest in the program. The desirable cholesterol cutoff point is 160 mg% for the children as recommended by Kannel (5). Several adult populations in the world, for example, Japan, have cholesterol levels in this range and have a lower incidence of this disease process (24). In the United States cholesterol levels rise with age (25). Thus a pediatric level below 160 mg% might give some future safety. An upper limit of 220 mg% is desirable for the adult, since in the young adult risk rises steeply when cholesterol

CHILDREN SCREENED FOR:

SERUM CHOLESTEROL
BLOOD PRESSURE
OBESITY
PHYSICAL FITNESS (ERGOMETRY)
CIGARETTE SMOKING

PARENTS SCREENED FOR:

SERUM CHOLESTEROL
BLOOD PRESSURE
OBESITY
EXERCISE HISTORY
CIGARETTE SMOKING
FAMILY HISTORY OF PREMATURE
    CORONARIES OR STROKES AND
    HYPERTENTION

Figure 6.   Coronary risk factors.

levels exceed approximately 200 mg%. According to the 25-year Framingham study, a serum total cholesterol is the best single chemical indicator of future risk (26). Our cholesterols are taken by finger-stick or venepuncture; we use only 1/20 mm of serum. The samples are taken nonfasting in the random state, since prior meal raises the cholesterol by only 3%. The test utilized is a direct colorimetric determination of Wybenga (Dow Chemical) (27). Figure 7 demonstrates the percentage of our families with a positive history of hypertension, premature coronaries, or strokes; percentage of children from 9 to 19 with elevated cholesterols; and percentage of parents who smoke—all significantly high.

Our cholesterol data. In our practice children's cholesterols at entry to the study rise with age—from birth to 2 months, 3 to 4 months, 5 months to 8 years, and 9 to 19 years. In the 9 to 19-year-old group, 35% of the children have cholesterols above 160 mg%. Other studies of pediatric cholesterol levels in the United States have shown even higher levels than ours (28). In our study as in others, there is positive correlation between children's and parents' cholesterols.

Blood pressure screening. Children's and parents' blood pressures are taken twice yearly beginning at the age of 3 to 4 and whenever the cholesterol determination is done. The blood pressure results are explained to the parents.

Obesity screening. Subscapular fat measurements are taken with a

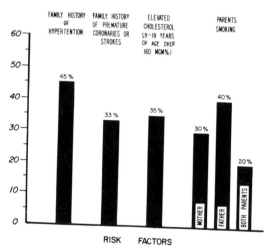

Figure 7. Scottsdale-University of Arizona longitudinal screening intervention program.

Lange skinfold caliper (29) beginning at 1 month of age and whenever cholesterols are drawn. The results are plotted on a nomogram (30).

Physical fitness in the child. A maximal index is computed after the child has pedaled to exhaustion on the bicycle ergometer. In this computation the child is compared to other children of similar ages in surface area (31). It is a sad commentary on our times that we are afraid to test adults for fear someone might suffer a coronary on this machine. Blood pressures and electrocardiograms are also taken with the ergometer test.

Cigarette smoking. The parents are questioned frequently about their own cigarette smoking patterns.

Three short-term community programs were developed as an outgrowth of our private practice program. Two small screening intervention programs were completed in two Scottsdale schools of fourth grade children and their parents over a 5-month period in 1971 and 1972 (Fig. 8*a* and *b*). Two other larger screening intervention programs were conducted by the Arizona Heart Association with a group of 220 children and parents in Phoenix, Arizona, and an equal number of fourth and fifth grade school children and their families in Bisbee, Arizona, a small southern Arizona mining community, both in 1972–73. In all of these programs there were four screening sessions that included measurements of serum cholesterol levels, blood pressures, skin fat folds, heights, weights, and exercise, and questionnaires about smoking and diet. The intervention program consisted of some in-school education and parent evening discussions. The purpose of these studies was to detect the number of families at risk and then attempt by education to reduce the risk factors. In each of these populations there were significant numbers of children and parents who were at risk and through these intervention programs it was possible to reduce these risk factors. However, through such short-term programs long-term adherence would seem to be very doubtful.

Arizona State Department of Health Nutrition Program

Beginning in 1972, the Arizona State Department of Health nutrition section under the direction of Anita Yanochik, R. D., began to incorporate this cardiovascular screening intervention program into their previously developed ongoing nutrition health delivery system, which has reached to date 10,000 Arizona preschool children and their parents through well-child clinics in several scattered communities throughout the state. The actual screening, which now includes cholesterols, blood pressures, smoking history, and other nutritional parameters, and the intervention are accomplished by trained nonprofessional aides living in these communi-

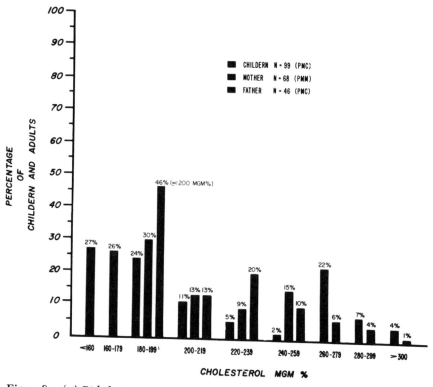

Figure 8. (a) Risk factor screening intervention, Scottsdale school study, 1971–1972, Pueblo Mohave Schools. (b) Phoenix "life underwriters" family risk factors.

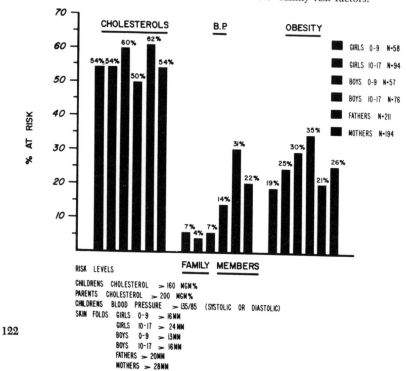

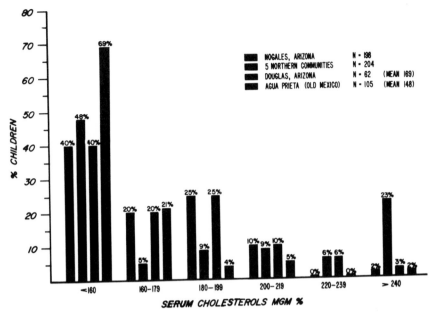

Figure 9.   Children's cholesterol levels in four Arizona areas and one Old Mexico area.

ties under the supervision of public health nutritionists. The results are gathered in a central computer facility. The cholesterol results utilizing the same micro-method of Wybenga are obtained in two central laboratories. The results of these screening endeavors in five northern counties in Arizona, the southern Arizona communities of Douglas and Nogales, and an old Mexico community cooperating in an international study in Agua Prieta are as follows (Fig. 9).

The subjects of the Douglas, Agua Prieta, and Nogales studies were 0 to 5-year-old children; children of all ages participated in the five northern counties. All were from fairly low socioeconomic groups. It was significant that the majority of the Arizona children had cholesterol levels above 160 mg%, many in very high ranges, whereas those in Agua Prieta were significantly lower (mean of 169 for Douglas versus 148 for Agua Prieta). The rate of cardiovascular disease in Agua Prieta, Mexico, is much lower than that of Douglas, Arizona, just across the border.

Cardiovascular Intervention Programs

The goals of our in-office and community intervention programs through behavioral change and long-term adherence are: to reduce the risk factors present in both children and their parents, and to prevent their future development in currently risk-free family members (Fig. 10).

GOALS: THRU BEHAVIORAL CHANGE AND LONG TERM ADHERENCE
 ● REDUCE RISK FACTORS PRESENT IN CHILDREN AND
   THEIR PARENTS

 ● PREVENT FUTURE DEVELOPMENT OF RISK FACTORS

Figure 10.   Family risk factor intervention program.

Our methods of intervention are shown in Fig. 11. We report all test results, for example, cholesterol, blood pressure, and ergometry levels, to the parents, with the associated desirable levels; we reinforce various segments of the program with each office visit by using free pamphlets and visual aids; we hold monthly evening parent slide presentations, which are also open to the community; we have an in-office nutritionist; and we have recently developed an alternative approach to the low-fat, low-cholesterol diet, which we believe may be desirable for long-term adherence (32).

Dietary Management

In our experience with children and young parents, who in general are not highly motivated, low-fat, low-cholesterol diets now recommended frequently fail to produce long-term adherence for three reasons: individual taste preferences are not respected; quantities of animal products rich in protein, fat, and cholesterol still tend to be excessive; and people have difficulty in remembering the cholesterol and saturated fat content of food even if they are interested in doing so. For these reasons we have found it easier to control the intake of cholesterol and saturated fat by limiting the animal protein intake to that of the recommended dietary allowances (RDA) (33), since the high-protein animal products generally also contain much cholesterol and saturated fat.

The basic concept is to limit the amount of animal protein to no more than that of the RDA (Fig. 12). (The average young American takes approximately twice the RDA for protein (15), mainly in animal products). As it turns out, if the protein recommendations are not exceeded it is difficult to get too much saturated fat or cholesterol in the diet. Values for the protein content of foods are given in a generalized form; for

 ● REPORTING ALL TEST RESULTS TO PARENTS
 ● REINFORCEMENT OF PROGRAMS WITH EACH OFFICE VISIT
   BY PAMPHLETS, VISUAL AIDS, DISCUSSION.
 ● MONTHLY EVENING SLIDE PRESENTATIONS.
 ● IN OFFICE NUTRITIONIST.
 ● DEVELOPMENT OF AN ALTERNATIVE APPROACH TO THE "LOW FAT
   LOW CHOLESTEROL DIET."

Figure 11.   In-office intervention methods.

DO NOT EXCEED RECOMMENDED DAILY
DIETARY ALLOWANCES (RDA) FOR PROTEIN
FROM MEAT OR DAIRY SOURCES

EXAMPLE :   ADULT WOMEN RDA = 46 GMS. PROTEIN
EAT NO MORE THAN 46 GMS. PROTEIN
FROM MEAT OR DAIRY FOODS.
(and may eat less)

Figure 12.   Basic protein-limiting concept.

example, one 8-oz cup of milk or 1 oz of cheese contains approximately
8 gm of protein, and 1 oz of cooked meat, fish, or fowl contains approximately 7 gm of protein (Fig. 13).

For example, the protein RDA for a 105-lb adult female would be 46
gm (Fig. 14), and no more than this should come from animal sources.
Thus 2 cups of milk or 2 oz of cheese contains 16 gm of protein and 4½
oz of cooked steak would have about 30 gm of protein and these would
supply all the animal protein necessary for this woman, and yet the

1 OZ. COOKED MEAT (includes fish and fowl) = 7 GMS. PROTEIN

1 OZ. CHEESE OR 8 OZ. MILK (dairy products) = 8 GMS. PROTEIN

Figure 13.   Average amounts of protein in animal products.

cholesterol content would be low (Fig. 15). For 16 oz of whole milk or 2
oz of cheese would contain 70 mg of cholesterol, and 4½ oz of meat
would contain 115 mg, giving a 185-mg cholesterol total for 24 hours,
much less than the American Heart Association's recommended 300-mg
cholesterol limit per day, and very much less than the average adult
American dietary intake of 600 mg. This diet would also be reduced in
saturated fat. It makes little difference what animal products are consumed, with a few notable exceptions such as eggs and organ meats,
which should be prudently reduced, and polyunsaturated fats should be

AGE (years)	GRAMS (protein)
1 – 3	23
4 – 6	30
7 – 10	36
11 – 14	44
MEN 23 – 51⁺ yrs.	56
WOMEN 23 – 51⁺ yrs.	46
PREGNANT	⁺30
LACTATING	⁺20

Figure 14.   Recommended daily dietary allowances (RDA) of protein (revised 1973).

ADULT WOMAN RDA = <u>46 GMS. PROTEIN</u>

EX. A DAILY EATING PATTERN

	PROTEIN (GMS.)	CHOLESTEROL (MGMS.)
16 OZ. MILK OR 2 OZ. CHEESE (2 X 8) =	16	70
4 1/2 OZ. MEAT, FOWL OR FISH (4 1/2 X 7) = ⌣	30	115
	46	185

Figure 15.   Calculation of dietary cholesterol intake by this *protein-limiting* method.

EGGS (USE SINGLY AND NOT DAILY) – YOLK
BUTTER, WHOLE MILK, CREAM AND ICE CREAM
LARD
LUNCHEON MEAT (BOLOGNA AND SALAMI)
ORGAN MEATS (LIVER AND BRAINS)
SHELLFISH (SHRIMP, LOBSTER AND CRAB)
COCONUT OIL (HIGH IN SATURATED FAT)
FATTY MEAT

Figure 16.   Use *sparingly* foods high in saturated fat and cholesterol.

- NON FAT OR LOW FAT MILK AND CHEESE
- MARGARINE (LIQUID OIL – 1 ST. INGREDIENT)
- FISH, FOWL (LOW IN SATURATED FAT)
- POLYUNSATURATED VEGETABLE OIL
- PLANT FOOD (VEGETABLES, FRUITS, BEANS, GRAINS AND NUTS)

Figure 17.   Foods low in saturated fat and cholesterol.

substituted for saturated fats (Figs. 16 and 17). It seems to make no difference by what method cholesterol or saturated fatty acid intake is reduced. The other advantages of this concept are that it allows for individual taste preferences; it is not wasteful, as excess protein yields only calories; it allows for easier maintenance of weight—animal products are rich in calories since they also generally contain much fat; it costs less by limiting expensive animal products, and this immediate advantage helps with compliance; it is easily adaptable to individual family eating patterns and to food purchasing; and it is easily explained by a nutritionist in a single consultation session. It probably is also adaptable to large groups of people (Fig. 18).

Hypertension Intervention

When blood pressures above 140 over 90 are detected in parents, they are encouraged to seek further medical care immediately. A significant number of our parent hypertensives were unaware of their condition until we tested them in our office. When the parents are hypertensive or if

● TASTE AND ETHNIC FOOD PREFERENCES ARE RESPECTED
● NOT WASTEFUL (EXCESS PROTEIN = ONLY CALORIES)
● EASIER MAINTENANCE OF DESIREABLE WEIGHT
● LOWER DOLLAR COST
● ADAPTABLE TO FAMILY EATING PATTERNS AND FOOD PURCHASING
● CONCEPT EASILY UNDERSTOOD

Figure 18.   Other advantages of the protein limiting concept.

there is a family history of hypertension, the excessive use of salt is discouraged in the infants' and children's diets, though salt is not restricted. Children in the upper percentiles of blood pressure are followed closely and we attempt to lower blood pressure by reducing obesity and increasing physical fitness. These latter suggestions, at least in adults, have been shown to have lowering effects on hypertension (21) and may lower blood pressures in children as well. Parents are advised of their own and their children's blood pressures in an attempt to keep them interested in this condition (Fig. 19a).

Smoking Intervention

The emphasis here is on frequent discussions with the parents about their own smoking problems (Fig. 19b). We discuss the possibility of harmful effects not only upon themselves, but upon their children as well. The latter emphasis seems to be having some beneficial effects in helping the parents change their own smoking ways. Several pieces of literature, concerning the health hazards of smoking, available from the American Heart Association, are given to the parents. Office smoking is discouraged.

Obesity Intervention

Here we attempt to help motivated obese children, but this is a difficult area and we obtain only limited success. Our major thrust is now in

● DETECTION OF HYPERTENTION IN PARENTS - REFERRAL FOR FURTHER CARE
● HYPERTENSIVE FAMILIES ⟶ DISCOURAGE EXCESSIVE USE OF SALT IN INFANTS
                          AND CHILDREN
● CLOSELY FOLLOW CHILDREN IN UPPER BLOOD PRESSURE PERCENTILES - THERAPY?
● ENCOURAGE PREVENTION AND TREATMENT OF OBESITY
● ENCOURAGE DEVELOPMENT OF PHYSICAL FITNESS
● REPEATED EVALUATION OF PARENTS SMOKING STATUS
● REPEATED DISCUSSIONS WITH SMOKING PARENTS CONCERNING HARMFUL
      EFFECTS ON THEMSELVES ⟶ THEIR CHILDREN
● "SMOKING" PAMPHLETS ARE DISTRIBUTED TO ALL SMOKING PARENTS
● IN OFFICE SMOKING IS DISCOURAGED
● PATHOLOGIC DEMONSTRATION OF LUNG CANCER

Figure 19.   (a) Hypertension intervention. (b) Smoking intervention.

- DEMONSTRATION TO PARENTS OF SUBCUTANEOUS "FAT" NOMOGRAM WITH EACH OFFICE VISIT
- INFANT AND CHILDREN EATING PRACTICES:
  - ENCOURAGEMENT OF BREAST FEEDING
  - DELAY IN USE OF SOLID FOODS IN INFANCY (4 — 6 MONTHS)
  - "LET APPETITE BE THE GUIDE" – THROUGHOUT LIFE
- EMPHASIS ON "EATING BEHAVIOR" RATHER THAN "DIETS"
- ENCOURAGE REGULAR AND ENJOYABLE PHYSICAL ACTIVITY
- DISCOURAGE NUTRIENT EXCESS
- DISTRIBUTION OF PAMPHLETS

Figure 20.   Obesity intervention.

the area of possible obesity prevention in the infant and young child (Fig. 20). The relationship of obesity to simple gross weight in the infant and child is unreliable. Consequently, we utilize the Lange skinfold caliper in measuring the subcutaneous fat in infants and children and by plotting the results on a nomogram which depicts the tenth, fiftieth, and ninetieth percentile of our population, we are increasingly able to interest mothers in this concept of obesity prevention.

The nomogram shown in Fig. 21 was developed from random values in our population prior to this intervention program. We hold discussions with parents about feeding practices in children and infants, and we encourage breast-feeding, delaying solid food (34), and allowing the

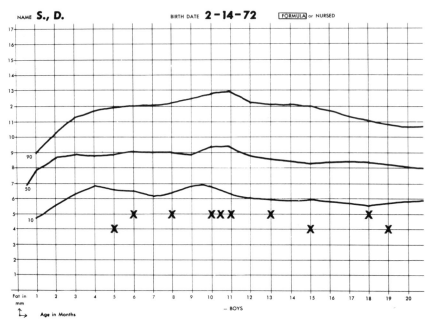

Figure 21.   Smoothed growth chart of fat tissue in males.

child's appetite to be the guide. We also encourage increased physical activity where applicable. Reprints and booklets are also distributed in connection with this risk factor.

Development of Physical Fitness

This is a difficult area of intervention. Family encouragement is given with each of the ergometer tests (Fig. 22) and each time the computer questionnaire is filled out, twice yearly. We suggest limiting television watching during the daylight hours. The older child is encouraged to learn carry-over sports so that he may become adept at a physical activity or activities that he can enjoy throughout his life. The frequency of the activity as well as its enjoyment is stressed rather than the type. Here, also, the parents are encouraged in this endeavor.

The cardiovascular intervention program of the Arizona State Health Department nutrition delivery system now has reached 10,000 families or 40,000 individuals in 10 counties, and for the coming year will involve another 13,500 families at a cost of $10 to $13 per family.

The initial screening performed by aides is accomplished in county well-child clinics. These results are also reported to the parents. When individuals at risk are detected, they are referred for appropriate medical care, but intensive individual nutrition counseling is also offered by these same aides in a home family setting, often with repeated visits in the hope of effecting change in the family's eating patterns. The "protein limiting" concept, which is acceptable to differing ethnic and socioeconomic groups, is also utilized in this setting. Advice is given about smoking and the other cardiovascular risk factors. Rescreening is performed at 6-month intervals. This entire program appears to be gaining acceptance throughout the state and is involving many sectors including University of Arizona College of Medicine, private medical practice, food industry, and local health departments, all cooperating to aid in its success.

● ENCOURAGEMENT OF FAMILY EXERCISE WITH EACH ERGOMETER AND CHOLESTEROL TEST

● ENCOURAGE PHYSICAL ACTIVITY IN INFANTS, AND CHILDREN

● PREVENT ACTIVITY RESTRICTION ●. g. T.V. DURING DAYTIME

● CHILDREN SHOULD LEARN "CARRY OVER" SPORTS

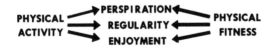

● DISTRIBUTION OF "PHYSICAL FITNESS" PAMPHLETS

Figure 22.   Physical fitness intervention.

In conclusion, we are dealing with an iceberg. The disease process and the risk factors have their inception in the pediatric age group where there is currently no significant screening or intervention. It is only when the problem emerges with the onset of a coronary or a stroke that we become concerned. By then, it is too late. We must start much earlier.

REFERENCES

1. J. Strong, *J. Atheroscler.* **9**: 251 (1961).
2. National Center for Health Statistics, Annual Summary, 1969.
3. H. C. McGill, Jr., ed., *Geographic Pathology of Atherosclerosis*, Baltimore: Williams & Wilkins, 1968.
4. W. E. Connor and S. L. Connor, *Preventive Med.* **1**: 49 (1972).
5. W. B. Kannel and T. B. Dawler, *J. Pediatr.* **80**: 544 (1972).
6. C. J. Glueck, F. Hechman, et al., *Metabolism* **20**: 597 (1971).
7. Data from the Health Examination Survey, Blood Pressure of Adults by Age and Sex, U.S., 1960–2, Reports from the National Health Center for Health Statistics, Publ. No. 1000, series 11, n. 4.
8. S. H. Zinner, P. S. Levey, E. H. Kass, *N. Eng. J. Med.* **284**: 401 (1971).
9. L. D. Dahl, *Am. J. Clin. Nutr.* **21**: 787 (1968).
10. Committee on Nutrition, American Academy of Pediatrics, *Pediatrics* **53**: 115 (1974).
11. Program Research Section, National Clearinghouse for Smoking and Health, U.S. Dept. of Health, Education, and Welfare, Rockville, Md.
12. A. J. Luquette, C. W. Landiss, and D. J. Merk, *J. School Health* **40**: 533 (1970).
13. P. Cameron, Kostin, et al., *J. Allergy* **43**: 336 (1969).
14. A. B. Palmer, *Soc. Sci. & Med.* **4**: 359 (1970).
15. Ten-State Nutrition Survey, 1968–70, Clinical U.S. Dept. of Health, Education, and Welfare Publ. No. (HSM) 72-8131.
16. L. I. Dublin and H. H. Marks, TR Life Insurance, M. Dir, American, **35**: 235 (1952).
17. W. B. Kannel, et al., *Circulation* **35**: 734 (1967).
18. C. G. D. Brook, K. Lloyd, and O. H. Wolf, *Br. Med. J.* **2**: 25 (1972).
19. J. Hirsch and J. L. Knittle, *Fed. Proc.* **29**: 1516 (1970).
20. National Adult Physical Fitness Survey, Newsletter President's Council on Physical Fitness and Sports, 14 May, 1973.
21. M. Fox and J. P. Naughton, *Amer. Heart Assn. Publ.* LI:17-20, April, 1972.
22. B. C. Johnson, F. H. Epstein, and M. O. Kjelsberg, *J. Chron. Dis.* **18**: 147 (1965).
23. J. L. Angel, *Am. J. Phys. Anthrop.* **7**: 433 (1949).
24. Report of Intersociety of Heart Disease Commission for Heart Disease Resources *Circulation* **42**: (1970).

25. Serum Cholesterol Levels of Adults, National Center for Health Statistics, Series II, No. 22, U.S. Dept. of Health, Education, and Welfare.

26. W. B. Kannel, M. J. Garcia, P. M. McNamara, and G. Pearson, *Human Path.* **2**: 129 (1971).

27. D. R. Wybenga, V. J. Pileggi, P. A. Dirctene, and J. DiGeorgia, *Clin. Chem.* **16**: 980 (1970).

28. G. M. Friedman and S. J. Goldberg, *J.A.M.A.* **225**: 610 (1973).

29. J. Mayer, *Human Nutrition*, Springfield, Ill.: Thomas, 1972, p. 328.

30. Unpublished results of subscapular measurements of American pediatric population 10, 50th, and 90th percentiles males and females.

31. S. J. Goldberg, *J. Pediatr.* **69**: 46 (1966).

32. G. M. Friedman, A. Yanochik, S. J. Goldberg, D. Bal, and N. West, *J. Nutr. Ed.* (in press).

33. Recommended Daily Dietary Allowances, Food and Nutrition Board, National Research Council, Revised 1973.

34. A. Shukla, H. A. Forsyth, C. M. Anderson, and S. M. Marwah, *Br. Med. J.*, **4**: 507 (1972).

PART 4

Control of
Childhood Obesity

10

Basic Concepts in the Control of Childhood Obesity

JEROME L. KNITTLE, M.D.

Department of Pediatrics,
Mount Sinai School of Medicine, New York, New York

Cellular studies of adipose tissue have demonstrated that the enlargement of fat depots in the extremely obese is due primarily to an increase in adipose cell number with varying increments in adipose cell lipid content (cell size). In general, subjects with a childhood history of obesity tend to display the most marked degree of hyperplasia whereas those whose obesity occurs after puberty have a greater contribution of adipose cell enlargement. In both cases, however, weight reduction is accomplished by alterations in adipose cell size without any appreciable effect on cell number. Similar results have been reported by other investigators who have confirmed the permanence of adipose tissue hypercellularity in obese adults even after marked degrees of weight loss (1,8,10,15).

Animal studies have also attested to the constancy of adipose cell number in adult life. One can restrict calories in the adult rat without altering cell number. As in man, the fat depot is depleted by changes in cell lipid content alone (7). Indeed only early caloric or protein restriction, or both, prior to weaning has been shown to decrease adipose cell number in the rat (9,13).

Thus both human and animal studies support the hypothesis that, in order to be effective in the treatment of obesity, dietary intervention must be instituted prior to the development of the hypercellular state. It is an all-too-common experience of the clinician to watch reduced subjects slowly reaccumulate weight after "successful" dietary programs have been ended. It is apparent that the reduced subject must continue to

135

restrict calories long after ideal weight has been achieved and perhaps for the remainder of his life. This latter fact may be due to the inability to lose adipocytes, and the metabolic consequences of altered metabolism in the fat cell of formerly obese subjects (10,16). In any event, the almost universal failure of obese subjects to maintain a reduced state indicates that a more rational approach to the problem lies in its prevention prior to the time of abnormal cellular and metabolic factors that predispose to and maintain the obese state.

In following this line of investigation over the past $3\frac{1}{2}$ years we have been studying obese and nonobese children ranging in age from 2 to 26 years. Adipose cell number and size were studied and the effects of three hormones (insulin, epinephrine, and growth hormone) on adipose tissue cellularity and metabolism were examined. This chapter summarizes the results of these investigations.

Body composition was measured either by determining total body potassium in a whole-body counter or by making calculations on the basis of height and weight using the Friis-Hansen nomogram (2,3,4,6). The correlation coefficient for ^{40}K and the calculated lean body mass (LBM) was 0.95, when used for subjects between the ages of 2 to 16 in whom the epiphyseal plate had not closed.

All obese subjects had a well-documented onset prior to puberty and were defined as individuals who were over 130% of ideal weight. Non-obese subjects were individuals with weights ranging from 90 to 120% of ideal. Individuals below 90% and between 120 and 130% of ideal weight were not included in this study. The ages of the subjects ranged from 2 to 26 years and the weights for obese subjects ranged from 28 to 175 kg. The youngest obese child studied was a 2-year-old girl who weighed 38 kg. Indeed, all obese subjects were above the ninety-seventh percentile for weight and height when plotted on Stuart's charts. Nonobese young adults over the age of 20 ranged in weight from 56 to 62 kg, whereas obese subjects of similar age weighed 97 to 170 kg.

At all age levels studied, obese children had, on the average, larger cells than nonobese children, although some degree of overlap was observed. However, it is significant that all nonobese children had cell sizes below adult values (that is, below 0.5 to 0.8 μg of lipid per cell), whereas the fat cells of most obese children had attained but had not exceeded adult values.

At all ages, obese children had a greater number of adipose cells. In one subject, age 6 years, the adult range was exceeded, and all teen-age subjects either attained or surpassed normal adult values. None of the nonobese children attained adult values before the age of 12. It would appear that in some obese children a rapid increase in cellularity begins between the ages of 5 and 7 years or earlier, whereas in nonobese children a similar occurrence is observed between the ages of 8 and 12, with little change in number between the ages of 2 and 8.

These results indicate that cellular development proceeds at a more rapid rate in obese subjects; indeed, deviations from normal development were observed as early as age 2 years. The data also suggest that by age 6 we can distinguish at least two subgroups within the obese population based on cell number: individuals with marked hypercellularity exceeding normal adult values, and those with modest increases in cell number relative to nonobese subjects of the same age but who have not exceeded the normal adult range. These subgroups can be further refined if we include differences in cell size. Thus there are individuals with marked hypercellularity who may have either increased cell size or normal cell size. Two similar groups can be identified within the obese groups with only modest elevations in number. The significance of these findings cannot be assessed at present, but they could prove to be an important basis for prognosis of childhood obesity. It is reasonable to assume that subjects who have exceeded normal adult values for cellularity will most likely retain their obesity, whereas those within the normal range or below may outgrow their "baby fat."

The data also indicate that fat depots of obese children develop in a quantitatively and qualitatively different manner from those of the nonobese. By age 2 obese children have larger cells as well as more fat cells than nonobese children. After that age there is a rapid proliferation of cells without enlargement in the obese subject that continues until about age 12 to 16. Nonobese subjects do not have significant increases in total fat until age 10, and then the increase is accomplished by changes in both cell size and cell number.

These differences in cellular proliferation were confirmed by longitudinal studies in the same individuals, studied at 1 and 2-year intervals. In these studies one sees more rapid and earlier proliferation of fat cells in the obese child at all ages, whereas significant increments in nonobese children did not occur until age 10 and older. It would appear that a critical period of adipose tissue development occurs somewhere between birth and age 2 and that this time period has important consequences for the future development of the size of the fat depot in the adult. A second period appears to be at the prepubescent and adolescent period, when cellular proliferation occurs again in nonobese subjects.

We have also studied the effect of weight loss on the increased cellularity found in our obese children. At all ages studied (18, 13, 11, 6, 5, and 2 years) decreases in body fat were accomplished by a reduction of adipose cell size without significant changes in cell number. Thus once a particular adipose cell number is achieved, whatever the age, one cannot decrease it by dietary restriction. However, studies of obese children under the age of 6 in whom cell number had not exceeded adult values indicate that one may be able to alter the rate of adipose cell development and therefore affect the ultimate number achieved as an adult.

Metabolic studies of these obese and nonobese children have included an examination of the effect of insulin, epinephrine, and growth hormone on adipose tissue cellularity and metabolism. Previous studies in adults have shown that adipose cell size plays a role in the sensitivity of adipocytes to insulin (16). The larger the fat cell the less sensitivity one sees when one measures $^{14}CO_2$ production from radioactive glucose. The larger cells from obese adults display less *in vitro* sensitivity than the smaller cells of nonobese subjects (50% increases over basal values versus 150 to 200%). However, this action of insulin appears to be secondary to the obese state and increased cell size rather than primary. Thus after weight reduction the smaller cells in obese subjects appear to respond normally. In addition, it has been demonstrated by Sims and associates that normal volunteers who have been overfed and increased in weight display an increase in cell size with similar *in vitro* insensitivity to insulin.

More recently we have shown that adipocytes from obese adolescents and children do not display *in vitro* insensitivity to insulin; we have further demonstrated in newly diagnosed juvenile diabetics that the *in vivo* effect of insulin in these subjects produces an increase in cell size without altering cell number (5,11). It appears that the action of insulin on the adipocyte is primarily one of maintaining or producing an increase in cell lipid content. Only in hypopituitary dwarfs treated with human growth hormone have we been able to demonstrate increments in adipose cell number that suggest a role for this hormone in cellular proliferation (14). Further studies are necessary, however, to clearly delineate the relative roles of insulin and growth hormone on growth, development, and metabolism of adipose tissue.

Another hormone of interest is epinephrine. We have shown a diminished response to the lipolytic effect of this hormone in cells derived from obese subjects regardless of age. After weight reduction this diminished response does not change. Since epinephrine is a major hormone in producing lipolysis in the fat cell it is tempting to postulate an etiological role in the development of the hypercellularity and increased cell size found in obese subjects. The fact that its action appears to be independent of age, cell size, and weight loss is further support for a primary role in the pathogenesis of this condition (12). Indeed if a genetic obesity does exist in man, it could manifest itself in the form of altered enzymatic activity.

One could speculate that the lack of epinephrine response serves as a stimulus for the development of new adipose cells. Thus a decrease in fatty acid released secondary to epinephrine stimulation could be overcome by providing a greater number of less responsive cells to meet energy needs. Since epinephrine acts through adenyl cyclase, one could also postulate a defect in this system. Studies of the levels of $3'5'$ cyclic adenosine monophosphate and adenyl cyclase in human and rat adipose tissue are currently in progress in our laboratory to explore this hypothesis.

In summary, the treatment of obesity in man has been largely limited to one form or another of caloric restriction after the development of the disorder. In general the success of these programs is measured by the amount of weight lost and the ease or speed with which ideal weight is achieved. Little, if any, attention is paid to the long-term consequences, which are almost universally disappointing. Our data clearly indicate that in childhood-onset obesity one should institute dietary regimens prior to age 6, or age 2 in some cases, if a lifelong history of obesity is to be avoided.

At present and throughout medical history the best treatment available to the obese patient has been weight reduction followed by the prospect of lifelong dietary restriction. The obese subject is exposed to a multitude of dietary regimens in both the lay and the scientific press that are merely one form or another of caloric restriction. They do not alter the natural history of the disease and are almost impossible to maintain. Obviously newer approaches are necessary if meaningful results are to be achieved. The early identification of abnormal growth and metabolism of fat depots coupled with therapeutic intervention prior to the attainment of the hypercellular state offers the best hope for the prevention and treatment of the obese state and its complications in both children and adults.

REFERENCES

1. G. A. Bray, *Ann. Intern. Med.* **73**: 565 (1970).
2. S. H. Cohn and C. S. Dombrowski, *J. Nucl. Med.* **11**: 239 (1970).
3. S. H. Cohn, C. S. Dombrowski, H. R. Pate, and J. S. Robertson, *Phys. Med. Biol.* **14**: 645 (1969).
4. B. Friis-Hansen, *Pediatrics* **28**: 169 (1961).
5. F. Ginsberg-Fellner and J. L. Knittle, *Diabetes* **22**: 528 (1973).
6. J. Hirsch and E. Gallian, *J. Lipid Res.* **9**: 110 (1968).
7. J. Hirsch and P. W. Han, *J. Lipid Res.* **10**: 77 (1969).

8. J. Hirsch and J. L. Knittle, *Fed. Proc.* **29**: 1516 (1970).

9. J. L. Knittle, *J. Nutr.* **102**: 427 (1972).

10. J. L. Knittle and F. Ginsberg-Fellner, *Diabetes* **21**: 754 (1972).

11. J. L. Knittle and F. Ginsberg-Fellner, Unpublished results (1973).

12. J. L. Knittle and F. Ginsberg-Fellner, *Clin. Res.* **17**: 387 (1969).

13. J. L. Knittle and J. Hirsch, *J. Clin. Invest.* **47**: 2091 (1968).

14. J. L. Knittle, L. Sussman, P. J. Collipp, and M. Gertner, Amer. Diabetes Assn. Meeting, 1972.

15. L. B. Salans, S. W. Cushman, and R. E. Weissmann, *J. Clin. Inv.* **52**: 929 (1973).

16. L. B. Salans, J. L. Knittle, and J. Hirsch, *J. Clin. Invest.* **47**: 153 (1968).

11

Behavior Modification in the Treatment of Childhood Obesity

HENRY A. JORDAN, M.D. and
LEONARD S. LEVITZ, PH.D.

Department of Psychiatry, School of Medicine, University of
Pennsylvania and the Philadelphia General Hospital
Philadelphia, Pennsylvania

The regulation of body weight in man is governed by an interaction between energy intake, energy expenditure, and the efficiency of the body's biochemical mechanisms. The input of energy is accomplished through ingestion of food, and the expenditure is the sum of muscular activity and the energy required by the organism to grow and to maintain its own internal state.

The body's biochemical efficiency determines the amount of useful energy derived from the energy supplied to it by ingestion. If this efficiency is high, relatively less energy is required to produce a physiological function. With the same amount of ingested calories and level of physical activity the organism with higher biochemical efficiency will have more energy available for storage in adipose tissue. Although the amount of energy utilized in maintaining many physiological functions can be measured, direct and significant alteration of biochemical efficiency is not possible at this time. Therefore, if we are to alter fat stores we must rely on producing changes in those factors over which we have

Work supported by Nutrition Foundation Grant No. 384, and by research grants MH-15383, Research Scientist Development Award (to Dr. Jordan) MH-37224, from the National Institute of Mental Health.

ntrol, namely, the intake of energy or the expenditure of energy through voluntary muscular activity.

While eating and muscular activity are behaviors which are under voluntary control, many aspects of these behaviors have become so habitual in the human adult that they appear to be automatic and involuntary. If, however, one looks at eating behavior in the newborn infant one can see how early parental teaching and attitudes begin to influence this behavior. For example, the breast-fed child sucks until satisfied and the mother does not know how much milk he has ingested. Physiologically, however, the mother produces milk according to the demands of the child. This important biological feedback system is completely disrupted when the breast is replaced by a bottle. Now the mother has a visual cue and can see how much milk the child has ingested. She can use this cue to shape the child's eating behavior according to her own attitudes about how much the child should eat. It becomes possible for her to overfeed or underfeed her child. Beginning with this process, the parent assumes a much greater role in teaching and shaping feeding behavior.

As a child grows, the range and complexity of behaviors involved in eating and muscular activity increase enormously. It is this set of complex behavior patterns, in interaction with the person's biochemical make-up, that governs the balance of energy and regulates the deposition of fat in the adipose depot. As each child has different genetic and environmental influences, so he develops different behaviors that enter into the regulation of body energy and weight. In most instances, these learned behaviors result in the regulation of normal body weight. However, Ullman (3) has outlined a number of ways by which a child may develop inappropriate eating habits that lead to disordered energy balance. For example, the child may learn to depend upon environmental cues for initiating eating. In the previous example of breast versus bottle feeding, the relationship between food delivery and the child's physiological needs is disrupted. As this occurs a child often is taught to rely on the cues provided by the parent rather than those provided by his own physiological needs. A common example of this process is the giving or withholding of parental approval in association with the amount of food remaining on the child's plate. Through repetition of this process, the cue for meal termination is no longer an internal satiety signal but becomes the act of cleaning the plate. In addition, food itself is a strong reinforcer since it satisfies physiological needs. Therefore, food may come to satisfy multiple emotional needs by being strongly and repeatedly associated with parental attention, comfort, and affection. Through this association, food may become a general way of coping with various emotional states. For instance, food can be used to reduce anxiety, alleviate pain, lift depression, relieve boredom, distract from loneliness, counter fatigue, or even enhance happiness.

Through eating in many situations and under a variety of conditions and experiences, ingestive behavior may come under the control of many influences other than those based on internal need. Not only may the parents actively teach inappropriate early behaviors and uses for food, but because the child patterns his behavior after that of his parents the eating behaviors of the parent become incorporated into the repertory of the child. It is through such behavioral developments as these that a behavioral component enters into the regulation of energy balance.

When a person maintains a stable body weight it can be assumed that a balance between energy intake and expenditure exists. It is often not recognized that an obese person, too, when maintaining a stable but elevated body weight, is maintaining a balance between intake and expediture. It is only during periods of active weight gain or loss that disequilibrium occurs. This disequilibrium may be a result of an alteration in biochemical efficiency alone. If the internal efficiency of the organism remains unchanged, however, there are three ways in which equilibrium can be disrupted so as to produce excess adipose tissue and hence weight gain:

1. intake of energy can increase while energy output remains unchanged;
2. intake can remain stable while output decreases; or
3. intake can increase and output decrease simultaneously.

Stunkard (7) described several syndromes, such as binge eating and night eating, in which ingestion of energy is clearly in excess of the energy requirements of the individual. On the other hand, Mayer (4) has shown that in many instances activity levels of the obese are clearly less than those of normal-weight persons. Most often we have observed both increased intake and decreased expenditure to occur simultaneously.

While these behavioral differences may account for weight gain, when weight stabilizes at either normal or excess levels, intake and expenditure are again in equilibrium. Even in states of excess adipose tissue, then, the behaviors involved in eating and activity are producing energy balance.

If we are to alter this equilibrium in order to create a negative balance and hence weight loss then we must influence these behaviors in some way. The traditional use of diets or exercise programs or both clearly is aimed at producing changes in behavior, but such changes are too often accepted in all-or-none fashion and patients soon become frustrated, give up, and return to previous behavior patterns. This happens with great regularity as people go on and off diets and exercise programs. What seems indicated are gradual changes in the behaviors that contribute to either high intake or low expenditure of energy. The changes must become part of the person's daily routine, and ultimately must be maintained by the patient himself.

During the past 6 years, programs aimed at producing behavioral changes in obese individuals have been devised and have shown promise in the treatment of obesity (6,8). This approach to therapy is called behavior modification and has been used in the treatment of a wide variety of psychological problems. In this treatment orientation, attention is focused on observable behavior and observed behavior change. The therapist and the patient are most interested in the specific behaviors that should be increased, decreased, eliminated, and instituted. To effect habit change, behavior modification attempts to abstract effective clinical techniques from general psychological principles of learning and motivation. Even if a behavior is partially determined by genetic or physiological factors, it can be altered or shaped.

In most disease states, whether physiological or psychological, we consider the problem to be a result of some abnormal functioning of the organism. For example, in diabetes one talks of abnormalities in glucose utilization; in mental retardation, about abnormalities in central nervous system structure and function. In disorders of energy balance, however, there is no clear distinction between normal and abnormal eating behavior or normal and abnormal activity patterns. Therefore, rather than label these behaviors as normal or abnormal, we must consider to what extent each particular behavior contributes to either an appropriate or an inappropriate energy balance.

In the treatment of obesity, behaviors that contribute to high intake of calories or low expenditure of energy are viewed as inappropriate and maladaptive. For example, eating nuts or popcorn while watching television (high caloric input–low expenditure of energy) is not maladaptive for a thin person but is clearly maladaptive for an obese person who is actually gaining weight or is trying to lose weight. The same can be said for the rapid ingestion of a piece of cheesecake while standing in front of the refrigerator.

In a behavior modification program the first step is to identify both appropriate and inappropriate behavior patterns together with the conditions that are associated with them. In order to do this, patients are required to keep written records of both feeding behavior and activity patterns.

The food intake record provides a way to continuously monitor human feeding behavior. Human feeding is an extremely complex behavior but can be viewed as having four major parameters. First, there is *ingestive behavior* itself, involving pace of eating, bite size, frequency of bites, pauses between bites, length of chewing time, and so on. On the food record we sample duration of eating to summarize these events. The second parameter is made up of *organismic variables* such as hunger, mood, and physical state of the organism. The third parameter is made up of *behaviors* that occur coincidentally with ingestion. In this regard, the person records his physical position while eating and any activities associated with eating. The fourth parameter is made up of *stimuli* preceding or concurrent with ingestion. Some of the most important stimuli are time and place of eating, other persons present during eating, and food characteristics such as type, amount, and caloric value.

In addition to recording the parameters involved in feeding behavior, patients also record two parameters of energy expenditure: the level of energy expenditure as indicated by the type of physical activity, and the place where the activity occurs. Recording is done at 15-minute intervals for the entire 24-hour period. During the first week of record-keeping patients are instructed to maintain their body weight and their usual eating and activity patterns.

After the completion of these records it is important to identify the behaviors that may be considered maladaptive. This is an essential task because a behavior that is maladaptive for one obese person may not be maladaptive for another. For instance, it has been suggested that the rate of eating is related to the amount of food ingested. While rapid eating may or may not be a habit that differentiates obese from normal-weight individuals, for some obese people this habit may account for a large part of overeating and may thus be maladaptive for appropriate energy balance. For other obese patients, however, a fast pace of eating may contribute only minimally to the problem of overeating with other behaviors being more important in accounting for the problem.

Incorrect assessment of the behaviors that are truly maladaptive will lead during treatment to random behavioral change, which will only serve to frustrate further both patient and therapist. Alteration of long-standing habits is difficult, and changing behaviors that do not contribute significantly to the disordered energy balance will not lead to weight loss.

Because this is such an essential step in this treatment approach we found it necessary to develop a precise method of analysis. Simply scanning the records to arrive at a clinical judgment of problem areas did not provide the precision required for a proper diagnosis. We have devised a self-analysis form on which the patient or clinician can summarize the frequency of ingestions that take place in conjunction with each stimulus, behavior, and organismic variable sampled on the food record. The analysis form acts as a marker or indicator for identifying areas that are not in keeping with the creation of a negative energy balance and hence weight loss.

From this form, for example, one might note that a high frequency of ingestions are occurring while the patient is alone. One would then look again at the food record specifically for those instances when the patient is eating alone. If the caloric value (amount or caloric density or both) of the food ingested while alone is high we conclude that eating alone is maladaptive for the patient. We have seen situations where this has been dramatically underscored: not only has caloric intake been high when ingestions occurred while the patient was eating alone, but intake was low when he was eating with others. This method of analysis is used for each parameter of eating so that the end result is a set of eating habits, each of which is maladaptive to the patient's goal of losing weight or maintaining weight loss. It is also important to note interactions among the parameters in order to specify the maladaptive habits precisely.

Once the entire cluster of components surrounding the maladaptive behaviors have been identified, specific recommendations and techniques for altering the maladaptive habits can be suggested to the patient. Although there are only a few general laws of learning, numerous therapeutic techniques can be derived from them. Selection of a particular technique must be based on the initial behavioral analysis so that there is a clear correspondence between the maladaptive habit and the technique chosen to effect the change.

Behavior change is often seen as an all-or-none affair: a person either eats dessert or he does not. One general principle of learning, however, is that behavior change proceeds most effectively by means of a series of small incremental changes, each step more closely approximating the final goal. In psychology this process is called shaping. From this general principle many specific techniques may be derived.

For example, an obese individual may habitually consume all the food on his plate regardless of the amount placed before him. The patient is using a clean plate as the signal for meal termination rather than using a signal based on some internal physiological satiety mechanism. The ultimate behavioral goal in reversing this maladaptive habit is to change the signal that indicates the end of the meal. It is unrealistic to expect the patient to change this long-practiced and automatic behavior overnight. Therefore, one utilizes the principles of shaping to devise a series of steps leading to the ultimate goal. The steps are programmed according to the patient's progress and designed to afford a high probability of success at each successive phase. The first step might be to leave over 1 teaspoon of food at the dinner meal. The frequency of the response and the amount remaining can then be increased over a period of time.

During the course of treatment a variety of techniques for changing the identified maladaptive habits are suggested. For example, the patient's food record may indicate a problem in the act of ingestion, such as eating too fast, taking large bites, or being generally unaware of amounts consumed. Techniques would be directed at teaching the patient to pause between bites, cut food into smaller pieces, delay between courses, and concentrate on the sight, smell, and taste of the food. The records may also show that eating occurs in connection with a side variety of stimuli, such as a particular time of day, being in a particular place, or seeing food. The patient should learn to confine his eating to a narrow range of stimuli. For example, he would gradually restrict eating to only certain times of the day and to one room of the house, and he would reduce visible food supplies through altered shopping, storage, and preparation habits. If the records show that many activities are associated with eating, such as watching television or reading, then the patient is instructed to do nothing else while eating. Organismic variables, such as fatigue, boredom, anxiety, and depression, may also precede overeating. These are perhaps most difficult to change, but programming alternative behaviors to eating may replace eating as a response to these emotional states.

After the patient is instructed in a behavioral technique, the record-keeping and analysis forms provide week-to-week feedback on changes he accomplishes in the target habits. By using the forms the patient is able to set realistic goals for a step-by-step change of behavior and then observe his progress toward his goals.

In a similar fashion one can devise techniques for increasing physical activity, which is as important as altering feeding behaviors in producing a negative energy balance. An obese and sedentary person will not be able to go out and run a mile or play a set of tennis; this would represent not only a physiological stress but an abrupt and major behavioral change. A better approach is to identify activities in which the patient currently engages and gradually increases both the frequency of these activities and the energy expended for each one. For example, the frequency and duration of walking may be increased by parking one's car further from one's destination, walking short distances instead of using mechanical transportation, or using stairs in place of elevators and escalators. All these changes, like those surrounding eating, can be accomplished in small, gradual steps.

The behavioral treatment program, then, is composed of a wide variety of techniques, each providing a partial change in the maladaptive habits of the obese patient. If these changed habits can be incorporated into the daily routine and life style of the patient and seen by him to be directly related to weight loss the chances of long-term treatment success are greatly increased.

Through this process of daily record keeping, weekly analysis, and slow change in both eating behavior and physical activity, the patient assumes responsibility for his own behavior, which must remain the ultimate goal of the treatment program.

The treatment of obese children with these techniques presents a unique opportunity to alter and shape behaviors as they develop rather than after they have become fixed in adult life. Until recently, however, behavior modification programs have been utilized only in the treatment of obese adults. At the Children's Hospital of Philadelphia preliminary work was conducted by Rivinus, Drummond, and Combrick-Graham to determine the feasibility and effectiveness of applying behavior modification to the treatment of obesity in children (5). This program attempted to answer the following questions:

1. Can preadolescent school children monitor their own behavior through record keeping and learn to use behavioral techniques for weight reduction?

2. Does the use of such techniques produce increased weight loss and lower drop-out rates than other more traditional treatment approaches?

3. What modifications in the adult program are necessary for application to the treatment of children?

Ten black children who were currently under treatment or awaiting treatment for obesity in an out-patient clinic at the Children's Hospital of Philadelphia were selected for study. The mean age of the seven girls and three boys was 10 years old (range 7–13), and the mean percentage above ideal weight was 70% (range 35–104%). A treatment team of a pediatrician, a psychiatrist, and a psychologist met with this group of children weekly for 10 weeks. Although the same records and techniques used with adults formed the basis of the program, three additional components were necessary. First, the children attended each session with their mothers or mother surrogates, and both were instructed in the procedures of behavior modification. Second, the treatment team and the subject group had dinner together at each meeting. These meals were eaten in the hospital cafeteria, which made it possible for the treatment team to model and reinforce appropriate eating behavior directly. Third, rewards were provided for the children contingent upon weight loss. In addition to providing motivation, rewards were chosen to encourage further adaptive behavior patterns. For example, rewards such as admission tickets to roller skating rinks or bowling alleys would produce increased physical activity.

These children were able to keep sufficiently detailed records on which to base treatment strategy. During the 10 weeks of treatment all nine children who continued in the program lost weight. The average weight loss was 6.2 pounds. These same children had gained an average of 3.5 pounds in the 10 weeks prior to treatment. During the program only one child dropped out of treatment, whereas previous experience in the outpatient clinic showed a 33% drop-out rate during a comparable time period.

An interesting sidelight was that the weight of the parent was closely associated with the child's weight loss. The four children whose mothers were obese lost an average of 2.6 pounds during treatment whereas the children of normal-weight mothers lost an average of 9.4 pounds. This suggests that active treatment of obese parents might be necessary to treat their obese child effectively.

Although no follow-up data are available the short-term results of this pilot study indicate that a behavioral approach to the treatment of childhood obesity is both feasible and promising.

Future programs should be directed at maximizing the effectiveness of this approach by determining which techniques are most suitable for children, which children and their parents are most suitable for this treatment, who might be the most effective therapists, and what follow-up procedures will enhance the long-term effectiveness of the program. In addition other settings, such as the school, with its personnel of nurses, teachers, dieticians, and physical education instructors, and accompanying facilities, may be more appropriate and effective than the hospital in treating obese children.

Many behavior modification programs for the management of other childhood behavioral disturbances have been effectively introduced to school situations. Furthermore, the training of nonprofessional therapists in the behavioral treatment of obesity has already been shown to be possible (2). Professionals such as teachers, who have not traditionally been involved in weight reduction, could be easily trained.

Another major area of further research is to assess the applicability of this therapeutic approach in altering parental behavior for the treatment and prevention of obesity. In treating preschool children who obviously cannot monitor their own behavior the parents must assume the responsibility of assessing and teaching their children adaptive eating behaviors and activity patterns. In the light of recent knowledge about the effect of early infant feeding on adipose cellularity (1) it becomes even more critical to investigate parental attitudes and behaviors in the first year of life. The results of such studies may provide cues for successful intervention in families with infants who have a high risk of becoming obese.

One of the difficulties encountered in treating an adult patient with long-standing obesity is that his maladaptive behaviors have been deeply overlearned and ingrained. These behaviors, then, have become resistant to change. The application of behavior modification to the treatment of obesity in childhood offers a unique opportunity to influence the development of adaptive behavior so that later the much more difficult task of eliminating maladaptive behavior will not be necessary.

REFERENCES

1. J. Hirsch and J. Knittle, *Fed. Proc.* **29**: 1516 (1970).
2. H. A. Jordan and L. S. Levitz. *J. Amer. Diet. Assn.* **62**: 27 (1973).
3. L. Krasner and L. P. Ullmann, *Behavior Influence and Personality.* New York: Holt, Rinehart & Winston, 1973.
4. J. Mayer, *Overweight: Causes, Cost, and Control.* Englewood Cliffs, N.J.: Prentice-Hall, 1968.
5. T. Rivinus, T. Drummond, and L. Combrick-Graham, Children's Hospital of Philadelphia Behavior Modification Program for the Treatment of Childhood Obesity. Unpublished manuscript, 1972.
6. R. B. Stuart and B. Davis, *Slim Chance in a Fat World: Behavioral Control of Obesity.* Champaign, Ill.: Research Press, 1972.
7. A. J. Stunkard, *Psychiat. Quart.* **33**: 284 (1959).
8. A. J. Stunkard, *Arch. Gen. Psychiat.* **76**: 391 (1972).

12

The Use of Hormones in the Treatment of Obesity

RICHARD S. RIVLIN, M.D.

Department of Medicine and Institute of Human Nutrition, College of Physicians and Surgeons, Columbia University, New York, New York

Hormones exert a variety of effects on intermediary metabolism, including that of lipids, and it is not surprising that they have been employed in the treatment of obesity. The reasons for the use of several hormones, their effectiveness, and the hazards resulting from their administration are reviewed briefly here. Particular attention is paid to thyroid hormones because they are the most widely used of the hormones in controlling weight, and because of the relatively greater risks associated with their use.

CHORIONIC GONADOTROPIN

Chorionic gonadotropin was used in the treatment of obesity by Simeons (1,2), who noted the similarity in appearance between certain obese patients and those with Frohlich's syndrome (3), a disorder characterized by sexual infantilism, overweight, and a hypothalamic or pituitary tumor. Patients with this disease presumably do not produce gonadotropin. A patient with this syndrome is shown in Fig. 1. Frohlich's syndrome is, in fact, very rarely a cause of obesity in childhood. Many children are obese

Research Supported by United States Public Health Service Grants AM-15265 and CA-12126, and by a grant from the Stella and Charles Guttman Foundation.

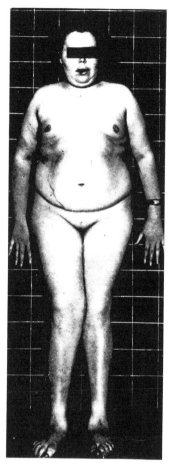

Figure 1. A 19-year-old patient with Frohlich's syndrome, illustrating the obesity and delayed sexual development that occur in this disorder (height age, 13–3; bone age, 14–0; FSH low; 17-KS: 0:5 mg/day; H.L.H. A22883). These patients presumably produce inadequate gonadotropin. Reprinted from Wilkins (3).

and appear to be sexually delayed, but most of them have no demonstrable pituitary abnormality and eventually mature normally (3). Nevertheless, Simeons treated a number of patients with daily injections of chorionic gonadotropin derived from urine of pregnant women, in combination with a 500-calorie diet, and reported short-term weight loss.

The considerable interest produced by these reports has resulted in a number of subsequent studies, both here and abroad. Carne (4) observed that in patients treated with chorionic gonadotropin on a double-blind basis, weight loss was not significantly greater than that observed in patients treated with daily injections of saline. He attributed the earlier results obtained with gonadotropin to the fact that the patients had received daily injections of some kind, a conclusion based upon his observation that patients who received daily injections of saline lost more weight than patients who received no injections at all.

Another investigator (5) suggested that the technique developed by Simeons was a satisfactory and safe method of reducing overweight patients in preparation for major surgery. In this report the patients were not studied in a double-blind fashion, and conclusions are difficult to draw.

In a recent summary of the accumulated literature to date, Gusman (6) claimed that chorionic gonadotropin appeared to be effective in causing significant weight reduction in approximately 60 to 70% of cases. The validity of this claim has been challenged by Albrink and the lack of adequately controlled studies has been clearly documented (7). A number of possible mechanisms of action of human chorionic gonadotropin have been proposed, including preventing hunger, elevating mood, causing euphoria, and producing redistribution of fat, but none has been proven by scientific evidence (7). It is possible that this hormone may have important effects on fat metabolism, or significantly influence hypothalamic-pituitary-gonadal function, but such hypotheses require experimental support. At present it seems unlikely that the administration of human chorionic gonadotropin is associated with any significant hazard to health, but even more unlikely that it is of significant benefit in the treatment of the usual case of obesity.

THYROID HORMONES

Because of the known effects of the thyroid hormones, thyroxine (T_4) and triiodothyronine (T_3), on accelerating metabolism, they have been suggested as a means of burning up the unwanted calories of obese patients. The widespread use of this method of therapy, and its possible hazards to health, require careful scrutiny. Although thyroid hormones have their many advocates, review of the published literature and consideration of the clinical effects of these agents suggest that their widespread application should be approached with caution and restraint for the following reasons:

1. Thyroid function is generally normal in obese subjects and there is no evidence that clinically significant hypothyroidism results from gradual weight reduction.

2. Thyroid hormones in doses commonly given will generally achieve variable degrees of weight loss, but only for the duration of hormone administration. Rapid regain of weight seems to occur following discontinuation of treatment.

3. The weight reduction that may be produced by thyroid hormones is inappropriate in that it consists of losses of significant amounts of nitrogen and calcium, with relatively little loss of body fat.

4. Administration of thyroid hormones may be associated with a significant hazard. The exquisite sensitivity of the heart to thyroid hormones must always be kept in mind in recommending their use.

To consider each of these points briefly, in turn, thyroid function tends generally to be normal in obese subjects, as determined by the conventional clinical and laboratory criteria (8,9). The reduced rates of basal metabolism that have been reported in obese subjects (10,11) may be more apparent than real, since calculations of basal metabolic rates are based on subjects in the normal weight range and may give misleading values in obese individuals (12). Values of uptake of radioactive iodine by the thyroid gland below 17%, which were considered low (10), may actually be normal (13) because of the increased dietary intake of iodine that now occurs in the United States. The significance of the shorter than normal biological halflife of T_3 and T_4 in obese subjects is still undefined, and the change in this parameter following administration of thyroid hormones may not necessarily imply a previously hypothyroid state (9,14). Decreased ^{14}C-T_3 recovered in adipose tissue from obese subjects at a single time point does not prove reduced accessibility of the hormone to peripheral tissues as has been suggested (9). The preliminary report (15) that thyroid hormone in serums from obese patients is bound to an abnormal protein has apparently not been confirmed by other investigators.

In a study of 26 obese patients Verdy (16) noted that all had normal thyroid function tests and that after they had fasted for 1 week there was an increase in the mean T_3 resin uptake but no change in the uptake of ^{131}I by the thyroid gland or in the total concentration of thyroxine in serum. The changes in thyroid hormone economy after fasting were not impressive.

In relation to thyroid hormone action in the obese, Bray (17) found that the activity of both the soluble and the mitochondrial α-glycerophosphate dehydrogenase in adipose tissue decreases with caloric restriction and that administration of T_3 prevents the decrease of the mitochondrial enzyme from occurring. The mitochondrial enzyme is known to be regulated by thyroid hormone and by dietary riboflavin (18). This hormonal mechanism could conceivably increase the metabolism of fat and result in increased heat formation during the treatment of obese subjects. The ultimate significance of this observation will depend to some extent upon greater understanding of the physiological role of the α-glycerophosphate cycle in health and disease.

The second reason for restraint in the use of thyroid hormones is that their effectiveness is transient. There is no doubt that under proper circumstances thyroid hormones will produce weight loss. Gwinup and Poucher (19), for example, using daily doses of either thyroxin or triiodothyronine for 30 weeks, noted an average weight loss of 25 to 30 pounds in their patients. Weight loss occurred only during the time that thyroid hormones were being administered, however, and one subject gained 28 pounds in 1 month after therapy was discontinued.

In a double-blind study, Hollingsworth and associates (20) noted that T_3 was effective in promoting weight loss in subjects on an 800-calorie diet, but only during the early phases of the study. When treatment was continued for 12 weeks the weight loss of patients treated with T_3 was no longer greater than that of controls, and following hospital discharge patients who had been treated with T_3 showed considerable degrees of weight gain. The fact that rapid regain of weight seems to occur with some frequency after cessation of therapy with thyroid hormones raises further questions about the long-term efficacy of this mode of treatment. The increase in appetite and the increase in food consumption that may occur in spontaneous hyperthyroidism, as well as in normal individuals treated with thyroid hormones, may initiate a habit pattern of food consumption that persists after the stimulus has been withdrawn.

Treatment of obese patients with thyroid hormones seems to be relatively ineffective when it is used on an outpatient basis (21–23), perhaps in part because of the difficulty in regulating food consumption. Goodman (23) noted that some degree of weight loss occurred initially with thyroid hormones, but after 1 year, obese patients who had been treated with T_3 had lost no more weight than those who had received placebos. In one out-patient study, treatment with desiccated thyroid appeared to augment the weight loss produced by amphetamines (24), but the long-term results after treatment ended were not reported.

The third reason for caution and restraint in the use of thyroid hormones in obese subjects is concerned with the nature of the weight that is lost. In an important study of body composition in two obese patients treated with thyroid hormone by Kyle and associates (25), measurements of body density indicated that the loss of mean body mass greatly exceeded that of fat. Loss of fat-free tissue rather than loss of fat was the major effect of thyroid hormone. The density of tissue lost in the two obese patients studied and in two patients with myxedema after each had

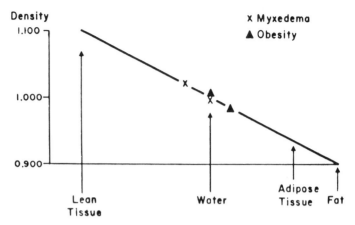

Figure 2. Density of weight lost by two obese patients and two patients with myxedema after each had received treatment with thyroid hormones. Shown for purposes of comparison are densities of lean tissue, fat, and adipose tissue. Adapted from Kyle et al. (25).

been treated with thyroid hormones is shown in Fig. 2. It is apparent that in both conditions the density of weight lost was considerably greater than that of pure fat or of adipose tissue.

These findings have been confirmed and extended, and in a recent study (26) breakdown of lean body mass accounted for nearly 80% of the weight loss produced by thyroid hormones. Thus only 20% of the reduction in body weight was attributable to a decrease in adipose tissue. Only in rare instances have reports appeared that did not show increased loss of lean body mass after treatment with thyroid hormone (27). In evaluating the effects of thyroid hormones, it is important to note that in obese patients who undergo caloric restriction alone, no change has occurred in lean body mass (28).

The loss of nitrogen is an undesirable side effect in the use of thyroid hormones in therapy. In addition to producing nitrogen loss, thyroid hormones tend to produce prominent increases in the urinary excretion of calcium. Data from Lukensmeyer and associates (29) bearing on this problem are shown in Table 1. In a group of normal adults, the urinary excretion of calcium was doubled shortly after treatment with large doses of triiodothyronine was begun. In children, whose calcium needs during growth are critical, any agent that depletes body stores should be viewed with caution. Results of animal investigations (30) suggest that thyroid hormone may accelerate the intestinal absorption of dietary calcium, but the relevance of this finding to growing children needs to be established.

The final problem posed by using thyroid hormones in the treatment of

Table 1   Urinary Calcium Excretion in Eight Normal Subjects Treated With Triiodothyronine[a]

Period (Weeks)	1	2	3	4	5	6	7	8	9
Treatment	—	—	—	T_3	T_3	T_3	—	—	—
Urinary Calcium	207	214	229	341	382	434	296	219	241
	±30	±24	±27	±34	±35	±44	±30	±23	±27
(mg/24 hr)									

[a] Eight young men aged 22–35 each received daily 400–500 μg of triiodothyronine in divided doses during the three 1-week periods shown. Adapted from W. W. Lukensmeyer et al. (29).

obesity is the hazard involved. Weight loss after the use of thyroid hormones is commonly associated with side effects. Gwinup and Poucher (19) achieved a mean weight loss of 25 to 30 pounds in their patients, as noted above, but with significant elevations in systolic blood pressure (6 to 9 mm) and pulse rate (18 to 25 beats/min), as well as nervousness, sweating, and palpitations. Some authors (9) have observed weight loss after treatment with thyroid hormones that appeared to be relatively well tolerated, but the majority of reports have described a number of untoward effects, often serious. The incidence of toxicity appears to vary widely among obese subjects treated with thyroid hormones (10). In one report angina was noted in 20% of adult patients treated (11). Tachycardia was noted in four of seven patients, and S-T segment and T wave abnormalities in five of seven patients treated with thyroid hormones in conjunction with total starvation (27). It has been suggested that some obese patients treated with large doses of thyroid hormones may not become particularly symptomatic, but they will nevertheless exhibit tachycardia and other metabolic responses (26). Thus, an obese patient who does not complain about the undesirable side effects of the thyroid hormones that he is receiving therapeutically may lead his family physician into a false sense of security about their safety.

The high frequency of cardiovascular symptoms in normal subjects after the administration of thyroid hormones is not surprising when one considers what is known about the metabolic actions of these agents. In an important early study Barker and Klitgaard (31) measured the oxygen consumption of the individual organs of the rat in response to the administration of thyroid hormone. As shown in Fig. 3, the oxygen consumption of the spleen, the brain, and the testes was not increased at all by thyroid hormones. The oxygen consumption of the remaining organs studied was increased to a variable degree, and was clearly increased to the greatest degree in the heart. The striking structural and functional effects of thyroid hormone on the heart have been amply confirmed and extended both

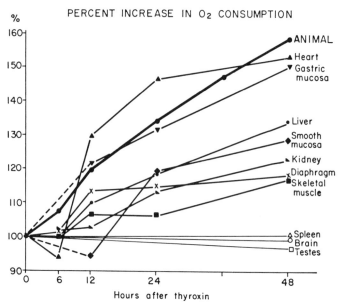

%   PERCENT INCREASE IN O₂ CONSUMPTION

Figure 3. Effect of administration of a single large dose of thyroxin on the rates of oxygen consumption of the individual organs of the rat. Results are shown in terms of percentage change with time. Adapted from Barker and Klitgaard (31).

in experimental animals and in man (32–34), and should always be kept in mind when prescribing thyroid hormones. In obese individuals in whom a greater burden upon the heart already may exist, the additional stress of toxic levels of thyroid hormone may represent a considerable risk indeed.

GROWTH HORMONE

Human growth hormone should be useful in many ways in the treatment of obesity. Growth hormone is very effective in mobilizing fatty acids and in depleting body fat. Acromegalic patients who have an excess of growth hormone generally have reduced body fat. The lipolytic effects of growth hormone are exerted without producing nitrogen loss, and in fact nitrogen retention is one of the hallmarks of growth hormone administration (35,36).

A detailed study of body composition in four male hypopituitary dwarfs before and after the administration of human growth hormone was reported by Novak and colleagues (37). Measurements were made for up to 18 months after initiation of therapy. It was noteworthy that despite rapid cellular growth and considerable increase in height and weight of the patients, there was no increase in total body fat during the first 12 months of therapy. During prolonged administration of growth hormone, and particularly when treatment was discontinued, a rapid increase in body fat resulted. Increase in linear growth and significant retention of nitrogen together with mobilization of body fat in 10 adult subjects treated with human growth hormone had been previously observed by Henneman and associates (38).

Further evidence for the potential value of human growth hormone in the treatment of obesity is the observation that this hormone has an intrinsic calorigenic effect (38–40). The effect is relatively small and its mechanism is not entirely clear. Increased calorigenesis is demonstrable in thyroidectomized rats (41), suggesting that growth hormone does not act by increasing thyroid function in experimental animals. This possibility has not been entirely excluded in man. Any agent that depletes body fat and increases energy expenditure without depleting nitrogen stores should be particularly welcome in the treatment of obese patients.

A study by Bray and associates suggests that growth hormone may be useful when administered in conjunction with triiodothyronine (42). The results of this study are shown in Fig. 4. When T_3 was given by itself to four obese subjects, oxygen consumption and nitrogen excretion were both substantially and perhaps proportionately increased. When growth hormone was added to the T_3 regimen, oxygen consumption increased even further, but nitrogen excretion was reduced to the control values. These investigators also noted that the diminished rise in plasma growth hormone concentrations in obese subjects in response to anginine infusion (43) could be increased towards normal by treatment with T_3 (44). This observation raises the possibility that the secretion of endogenous growth hormone and its consequent metabolic actions might also be increased by T_3.

Questions remain concerning the long-term efficacy of growth hormone administration to obese subjects and the likelihood that resistance or complications will develop with prolonged use. At present supplies of human growth hormone are extremely limited. It is unfortunate that unlike insulin, growth hormone from sheep, pigs, and cattle is ineffective in man (36). One must raise the ethical consideration of whether the precious amounts of human growth hormone should be used to treat a disease for which other means of therapy are available, when such use would necessitate restricting the availability of growth hormone to those growth-retarded hypopituitary children for whom no other therapy is effective. The planning of treatment for large groups of patients must be based on the availability of medical resources as much as on theoretical metabolic considerations.

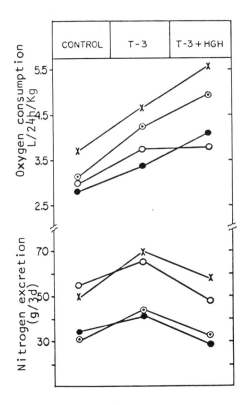

Figure 4. Effect of administration of triiodothyronine (T_3), and T_3 together with human growth hormone, on the rates of oxygen consumption and the magnitude of nitrogen excretion in four obese subjects. Adapted from Bray et al. (42).

PROGESTERONE

Hormones may be useful in the treatment of certain specific complications of obesity. It is well known that certain obese patients suffer from alveolar hypoventilation. This condition is believed to be due to the increased mass of the chest wall, increased intraabdominal pressure, and decreased expiratory reserve volume of the lung (45,46). The administration of progesterone has been of value in obese patients with hypoventilation in increasing the tidal volume (47), thereby ameliorating the respiratory acidosis and increasing the oxygen content of peripheral blood. It is not entirely clear how progesterone stimulates ventilation or how this effect is related to other metabolic actions of progesterone.

CONCLUSIONS

Hormones exert important roles in intermediary metabolism. Knowledge about their physiological functions has expanded in recent years but remains incomplete. Theoretical aspects and practical applications of several of the hormones employed in the treatment of obesity have been reviewed. But the problem of obesity remains complex and multifactorial. At present hormones should be used with caution and restraint. The potential usefulness of hormones in the therapy of childhood obesity will require continuing evaluation as new knowledge is acquired about basic mechanisms of hormone action.

REFERENCES

1. A. T. W. Simeons, *Lancet* **2**: 946 (1954).
2. A. T. W. Simeons, *J. Am. Ger. Soc.* **4**: 36 (1956).
3. L. Wilkins, *The Diagnosis and Treatment of Endocrine Disorders in Children and Adolescence*, 3rd ed., Springfield, Ill.: Thomas, 1965, pp. 262–263.
4. S. Carne, *Lancet* **2**: 1281 (1961).
5. P. Lebon, *J. Am. Ger. Soc.* **9**: 998 (1961).
6. H. A. Gusman, *Am. J. Clin. Nutr.* **22**: 686 (1969).
7. M. Albrink, *Am. J. Clin. Nutr.* **22**: 681 (1969).
8. C. Mautalen and R. W. Smith, Jr., *Am. J. Clin. Nutr.* **16**: 363 (1965).
9. J. L. Rabinowitz and R. M. Myerson, *Metabolism* **16**: 68 (1967).
10. E. S. Gordon, M. Goldberg, and G. J. Chosy, *J.A.M.A.* **186**: 50 (1963).
11. E. J. Drenick and J. L. Fisher, *Curr. Therap. Res.* **12**: 570 (1970).
12. S. C. Werner, Ed., *The Thyroid*, 2nd ed., New York: Harper & Row, 1962, pp. 129–140.
13. J. A. Pittman, G. E. Dailey, and J. R. Beschi, *N. Engl. J. Med.* **280**: 1431 (1969).
14. F. L. Benoit and F. Y. Durrance, *Am J. Med. Sci.* **249**: 647 (1965).
15. I. B. Perlstein, B. N. Premachandra, and H. T. Blumenthal, *J. Clin. Invest.* **45**: 1056 (1966) (abstract).
16. M. Verdy, *Canad. Med. Assn. J.* **22**: 1031 (1968).
17. G. Bray, *J. Clin. Invest.* **48**: 1413 (1969).
18. G. Wolf and R. S. Rivlin, *Endocrinology* **86**: 1347 (1970).
19. G. Gwinup and R. Poucher, *Am. J. Med. Sci.* **254**: 416 (1967).
20. D. R. Hollingsworth, T. T. Amatruda, Jr., and R. Scheig, *Metabolism* **19**: 934 (1970).
21. D. Adlersberg and E. Mayer, *J. Clin. Endocr.* **9**: 275 (1949).
22. D. A. W. Edwards and G. M. Swyer, *Clin. Sci.* **9**: 115 (1950).
23. N. G. Goodman, *Med. Ann. D.C.* **38**: 658 (1969).
24. N. M. Kaplan and A. Jose, *Am. J. Med. Sci.* **260**: 105 (1970).

25. L. H. Kyle, M. F. Ball, and P. D. Doolan, *N. Engl. J. Med.* **275**: 12 (1966).

26. G. A. Bray, K. E. W. Melvin, and I. J. Chopra, *Am. J. Clin. Nutr.* **26**: 715 (1973).

27. G. Sabeh, J. V. Bonessi, M. E. Sarver, C. Moses, and T. S. Danowski, *Metabolism* **14**: 603 (1965).

28. J. E. Christian, L. W. Combs, and W. V. Kessler, *Am. J. Clin. Nutr.* **15**: 20 (1964).

29. W. W. Lukensmeyer, J. H. Hege, G. B. Theil, and W. R. Wilson, *Am. J. Med. Sci.* **259**: 282 (1970).

30. D. M. Taylor, *Experientia* **24**: 837 (1968).

31. S. B. Barker and H. M. Klitgaard, *Am. J. Physiol.* **170**: 81 (1952).

32. R. Bressler and B. Wittels, *J. Clin. Invest.* **45**: 1326 (1966).

33. C. K. Friedberg, *Diseases of the Heart*, 3rd ed., Philadelphia: Saunders, 1966, pp. 1609–1628.

34. S. C. Werner and S. H. Ingbar, eds., *The Thyroid*, 3rd ed., New York: Harper & Row, 1971, pp. 551–560.

35. S. C. Woods, E. Decke, and J. R. Vasselli, *Psychological Reviews*, in press, 1973.

36. R. L. Ney, in *Duncan's Diseases of Metabolism*, 6th ed., P. K. Bondy and L. E. Rosenberg, Eds., Philadelphia: Saunders, 1969, pp. 721–725.

37. L. P. Novak, A. B. Hayles, and M. D. Cloutier, *Mayo Clin. Proc.* **47**: 241 (1972).

38. P. H. Henneman, A. P. Forbes, M. Moldawer, E. F. Dempsey, and E. L. Carroll, *J. Clin. Invest.* **39**: 1233 (1960).

39. H. S. Soroff, R. R. Rozin, J. Mooty, J. Lister, and M. S. Raben, *Ann. Surg.* **166**: 739 (1967).

40. G. A. Bray, *J. Clin. Endocr.* **29**: 119 (1969).

41. E. S. Evans, M. E. Simpson, and H. M. Evans, *Endocrinology* **64**: 836 (1958).

42. G. A. Bray, M. S. Raben, J. Londono, and T. F. Gallagher, Jr., *J. Clin. Endocr.* **33**: 293 (1971).

43. P. Beck, J. H. T. Koumans, C. A. Wintering, F. Stein, W. H. Daughaday, and D. M. Kipnis, *J. Lab. Clin. Med.* **64**: 654 (1964).

44. J. H. Londono, T. F. Gallagher, Jr., and G. A. Bray, *Metabolism* **18**: 986 (1969).

45. C. S. Burwell, E. D. Robin, R. D. Whaley, and A. G. Bickelmann, *Am. J. Med.* **21**: 811 (1956).

46. B. J. Kaufman, M. H. Ferguson, and R. M. Cherniak, *J. Clin. Invest.* **38**: 500 (1959).

47. H. A. Lyons and C. T. Huang, *Am. J. Med.* **44**: 881 (1968).

13

Behavioral Correlates
of the Obese Condition

M.R.C. GREENWOOD, Ph.D.
Institute of Human Nutrition, College of Physicians and Surgeons,
Columbia University, New York, New York

and PATRICIA R. JOHNSON, Ph.D.
Department of Biology, Vassar College, Poughkeepsie, New York

Obesity is not a disorder with a single cause. Although the normal regulation of adipose tissue mass is clearly in disarray in a clinically obese subject, the etiology of the regulatory dysfunction is far from understood. A number of studies have provided data on the metabolic and morphological factors associated or correlated with obesity (1,2,3,4). Nonetheless, whether one considers the increased caloric intake or decreased activity as behaviors that precede or that follow metabolic changes in the organism, the behavioral correlates of obesity are worthy of attention by those interested in analyzing this very complex disease state. Although the repertoire of behaviors that can be utilized by any organism to regulate its caloric intake and output are numerous and of varying degrees of subtlety, they fall into two general categories: behaviors associated with ingestion and behaviors associated with activity.

BEHAVIORAL CORRELATES OF INGESTION IN NORMAL AND EXPERIMENTALLY OBESE ANIMALS

In the study of body weight regulation and its abnormalities, numerous laboratory animal models have been used, including goats (5,6), dogs (7),

163

monkeys (9) and cats (9). The most commonly employed animal model, however, is still the albino rat. Since the discovery that bilateral electrolytic destruction of the centromedial nucleii of the hypothalamus produces hyperphagia and obesity (10), the classic preparation for studying normal body weight regulation and obesity has been the ventromedial hypothalamically (VMH) lesioned rat and its normal control.

The normal animal is responsive to many cues that guide its caloric intake behavior. These cues have been described as internal (physiological) or external (influenced by the environment). Internal cues include not only metabolites produced before and after ingestion, and hormonal signals that vary with absorptive state, but also factors such as gastric distention (11). External cues are mediated by gustatory, olfactory, and visual inputs to the central nervous system. There is evidence that under normal conditions the taste, sight, and smell of food are involved in body weight regulation. For example, although normal rats can, after a learning period, maintain body weight by intragastric injection of their diet (12), they do it much more effectively when injections are accompanied by oropharyngeal cues (13). In normal animals manipulating external cues, for example, increasing or decreasing the palatability or the odor of the diet, results in the expected ingestive response. Rats eat more of a palatable and less of a nonpalatable diet upon brief exposure, but adjust caloric intake appropriately if long-term feeding is introduced.

Le Magnen (14,15) has demonstrated and Kissileff (16) has also suggested that in rats the postmeal interval is highly correlated with the preceeding meal size. Furthermore, if caloric requirements change, there is a long latency before the animal changes the size or frequency of its meals. The control of meal size and frequency could therefore act as a long-term regulatory mechanism and is influenced by external cues and learned behaviors. Rats made obese by electrolytic destruction of their ventromedial hypothalamus display aberrant food-motivated behaviors. Lesioned rats become hyperphagic and gain weight to reach levels more than twice that of controls (9). However, in spite of elevated ad libitum intake, when lesioned animals are presented with the operant task of having to increase the number of bar presses to obtain a pellet of food, they perform less well than normal rats. Since the ability to increase the number of presses necessary to maintain food intake has been suggested as a measure of "hungriness" (17), that is, the hungrier the normal rat the harder he works, one would have to conclude on the basis of this test that lesioned obese rats and mice were less hungry than normal rats. This, then, leaves the paradoxical situation of an animal that eats voraciously ad libitum, but is not motivated sufficiently to perform work to obtain food. Furthermore, it has been reported that lesioned rats are more sensitive to quinine adulteration of liquid (18) or solid (7,19) diet and adapt less well to caloric dilution (18) than normal rats. These behaviors have been referred to collectively as "finickiness" (18). Lesioned rats have also been reported to show disruptions in the normal diurnal feeding pattern (20).

BEHAVIORAL CORRELATES OF INGESTION IN GENETICALLY OBESE RATS

The use of the VMH lesioned rat as a model for human obesity has provided much insight into the neural regulation of ingestion. One might, however, ask if the syndrome described in the VMH lesioned rat is characteristic of naturally occurring obesities. We investigated this possibility using the genetically obese Zucker rat (fafa), its VMH lesioned lean littermate, and its lean littermate. Using the classic procedures of Teitelbaum (21), we were able to show that when genetically obese rats were asked to press a bar for food on increasingly difficult schedules they performed as well as or better than their normal lean littermates. The VMH lesioned littermate showed the classic decreasing response pattern (Fig. 1) described by many others (22). Another series of experiments demonstrated that when the food of Zucker obese, lean, and VMH lesioned rats was adulterated with quinine, the obese and lean animals responded in a similar fashion and unlike the VMH lesioned rat (23). The obese and lean rats maintained caloric intake on higher levels of quinine than the VMH lesioned rats (Fig. 2). These data point to the conclusion that gross hypothalamic dysfunction, equivalent to electrolytic destruction of a part of the hypothalamus, is not an inevitable correlate of obesity. It is not clear what more subtle alterations in hypothalamic functioning might be present, but clearly hyperphagia and obesity can occur without the "unwillingness to work" or "finickiness" syndrome.

There are numerous more subtle interactions that could provide partial explanations. For example, Pfaff (4) was able to correlate nucleolar size (presumably indicative of increased ribosomal formation) in cells of ventromedial nuclei with the nutritional status of his rats. The ventromedial neuronal nucleoli of well-fed rats were larger than nucleoli in similar cells of underfed rats. These data lead to the conclusion that alterations in cellular protein synthesis in VMH lesioned rats may result from ordinary dietary manipulations. Evidence that some cells in the central nervous system may respond directly to dietary manipulation by changes related to protein-synthesizing activity, while other cells show no such response, points to at least one way that a genetic mutation could affect

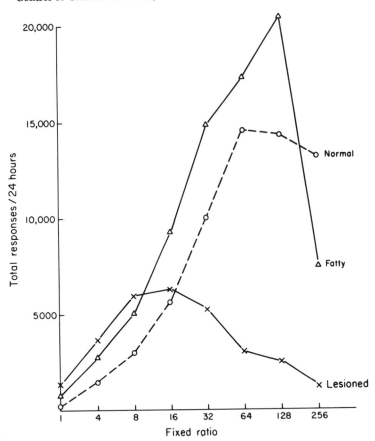

Figure 1. The effect of increasing workload on performance of obese (fafa), lean, and VMH lesioned lean Zucker rats. From Greenwood et al. (22).

the central nervous system and its body weight regulating function. One might hypothesize a regulatory error in which certain cells of the ventromedial hypothalamus were incapable of the appropriate quantitative response to input signals generated by caloric intake. The altered cellular response might, in turn, lead to alterations in ingestive behavior.

Another less obvious influence on the VMH lesioned rat could involve a regulatory error in the interpretation of orogastric cues. Rats presented with a highly palatable diet make moderate errors in intake, suggesting that there are reinforcing components associated with the orosensory signals generated by the food during ingestion (15). If the appropriate sensing of excess caloric intake were absent, or moderately altered, this reinforcement could presumably be a sufficient stimulus to continue in-

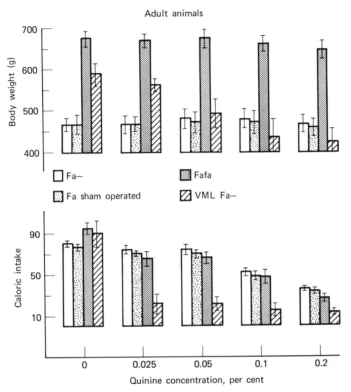

Figure 2. Mean body weight and caloric intake as a function of quinine adulteration for groups of adult rats as follows: normal, sham operated, genetically obese, and VMH lesioned. (There were six subjects in each group. Abbreviations: Fa — = non-obese; fafa = genetically obese; VML = ventromedial hypothalamic lesioned.) From Cruce et al. (23).

gestion. Subtle changes in neuronal metabolism of VMH lesioned rats resulting from alterations in protein-synthesizing activity and the incorrect modulation of orosensory cues are both mechanisms that could be involved as partial explanations for regulatory errors in caloric intake made by human subjects who show no gross VMH pathology.

BEHAVIORAL CORRELATES OF INGESTION IN HUMANS

The syndrome seen in the VMH lesioned rat has been extrapolated to the human condition by Schachter and his colleagues, and has gained considerable popular attention. Although provocative, the externality theory of Schachter fails to provide a completely satisfactory explanation for many crucial experimental observations. Schachter (25) and Nisbett (26) performed a number of experiments with obese humans from which they concluded that obese humans behave like rats made obese by VMH lesions. In the Schachter and Nisbett comparison, both VMH lesioned rats and obese humans are more sensitive to external than to internal cues; that is, VMH rats are "finicky" and will not work for food, and obese humans behave in the following ways: if food is readily (27) or attractively available (28) or is presented at an appropriate time to eat (25), the obese are much more likely than normal weight individuals to consume it. If instead food is harder to obtain, for example, if the subject must walk to a refrigerator or shell nuts, the obese are less likely to consume food (27). An additional experiment suggested that quinine adulteration of food had a proportionally greater effect on the obese than on normal weight subjects (29). Experiments by others (30) had previously suggested that some obese individuals were unable to adjust intake appropriately when liquid diets were diluted and the amount of intake could not be monitored with the use of visual cues. Although internal gastric cues are currently considered of minor importance in the human, it should be noted that some obese individuals have considerably more difficulty than some normal weight subjects when asked to report gastric contractions (30).

Schachter and colleagues presented the hypothesis that obese humans either do not, or cannot, pay attention to the normal internal physiological mechanisms that monitor hunger and satiety, but rather are cued by external factors in their environment. In their analogy, the obese human displays both the ad libitum hyperphagia characteristic of the VMH lesioned rat and the "unwillingness to work" syndrome.

Attempts to assess this hypothesis experimentally have not been satisfactory. Some of the difficulties may derive from the fact that experimenters have used very different subject populations. The obese subjects in different studies vary from 20 to 200% over ideal body weight and the age of onset of obesity is not always noted. Evidence is continually accruing to suggest that numerous subgroups exist in the obese population. One can distinguish between human obesities on the basis of metabolic abnormalities, adipose depot morphology, degree of overweight, and age of onset of obesity. In addition, distinctions are now being made on the basis of behavior, and these distinctions may in some cases correlate with subgroups defined by metabolic, morphologic, or developmental criteria. For example, testing procedures have indicated that juvenile-onset obese individuals experience distortions in perception of their body image (Fig. 3) and become extremely depressed (31,32) during weight reduction,

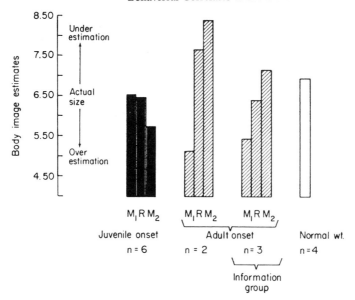

Figure 3. Body size perception of juvenile- and adult-onset obese subjects and of normal-weight subjects. Two sets of columns for the adult-onset subjects show perceptions when no information was supplied (left) and when they were permitted to view themselves in a mirror. M_1 refers to initial maintenance period in the hospital, R is the induction period, and M_2 is the final maintenance at lower weight period. From J. Grinker, *J. Amer. Diet. Assoc.* **62**: 30 (1973).

symptoms reminiscent of those seen during starvation. In adult-onset obese, the persistent symptoms of depression are absent. Timing behavior was similarly affected, with juvenile-onset obese showing changes in timing perception whereas adult-onset obese did not (33). These findings in juvenile-onset obese tend to support earlier psychogenic theories that would correlate long-standing obesity with childhood and adolescent experience and the development of distorted personality constellations.

A repetition of Schachter's "cracker" experiment using as subjects obese individuals who compare well with lesioned rats in respect to percentage overweight, that is, 100 to 150% over ideal body weight, failed to demonstrate the inability of the subjects to respond to a preload by selectively suppressing intake. Furthermore, there were no demonstrable effects among the subgroups of obese tested (34); that is, the adult-onset and the juvenile-onset obese responded similarly (Fig. 4).

Experiments designed with appropriate psychophysical procedures that tested taste thresholds, taste preference, and response to other external cues established that grossly obese (40% above ideal body weight) individuals were within normal limits with respect to detectability of sucrose

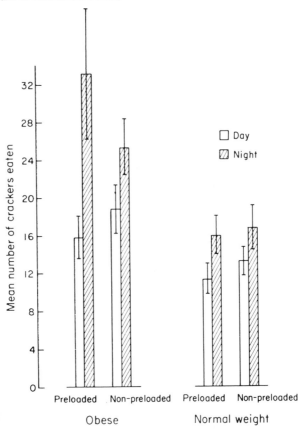

Figure 4. Number of crackers eaten by obese and normal-weight subjects as a function of deprivation condition and time of testing. (Values represent $\bar{X}$ and SE_M.) From Price and Grinker (34).

solutions, were no more biased than normal subjects by the addition of a red cherry color (Fig. 5), but preferred lower concentrations of sucrose solutions than normal-weight individuals (35), suggesting that the grossly overweight subjects were not more externally cued in the carefully controlled testing situation. One long-term study of caloric regulation has shown that at least some obese individuals compensate for caloric variability as well as normal-weight controls, although in both normal and obese subjects, regulation in response to dilution is lengthy and sometimes incomplete (36).

It is not surprising that some investigators disagree with the Schachter hypothesis that the obese human is responding like the VMH lesioned rat. In only the rarest cases of human obesity have gross abnormalities of

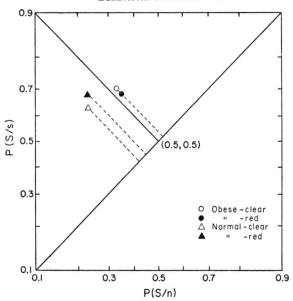

Figure 5. Estimates of response bias for obese and normal weight subjects in the red and clear color conditions. From Grinker et al. (35).

the hypothalamus been reported. It is even less surprising that the VMH lesioned rat does not provide an entirely adequate model for the study of human obesity when one analyzes the lesioned animal's syndrome more closely. That the hypothalamus plays a major role in the regulation of body weight can hardly be disputed, but the exact delineation of its role remains undetermined. It is now known that the exact site of the lesion (37), the size of the lesion (38), and the type of electrode used for lesioning (39) all affect the degree of expression of the obese syndrome. Furthermore, knife cuts as well as lesions produce hyperphagia and obesity (40). Additionally, electrically elicited hyperphagia from stimulation of lateral hypothalamic areas has been described as nondiscriminating (41); that is, gnawing and eating-like behavior can be extended to nonfood items, suggesting the production of a diffuse behavior that results in ingestion when food is present. Lesions placed in other areas of the brain, especially but not exclusively in the limbic area, will also produce food-directed behaviors (42). Evidence is also available that stimulation of areas outside the lateral hypothalamus also elicits an anorexic response in rats (42).

Further support for the idea that the hypothalamic system must be complex and hierarchal comes from the observations that VMH lesioned rats do regulate their body weight even though at higher than normal levels. Hoebel and Teitelbaum (43) showed that when rats are made obese preoperatively and then ventromedially lesioned, the rats will initially lose some weight; however, they remain obese and regulate around this elevated body weight. Reciprocally, Powley and Keesey (44) have reported that when prelesioned rats have their body weight and therefore their adipose depots reduced before lesioning of the lateral hypothalamus, they recover the ability to regulate body weight more quickly than control rats, but regulate at a lower level.

So far the available data continue to support the concept proposed by Stellar (45) that the hypothalamus acts as the mediator of internal and external central inputs, but do not exclude the possibility of other major control areas that may be activated by pathological disturbance.

As encephalization increases it is reasonable to expect that higher centers have certain "override" potentials. As suggested by Hirsch's model (46) and Jacobs's hypothesis (19), the importance of higher center influence may be not only in determining whether an animal eats, but the manner or mode of eating that is displayed. In pathologies such as obesity or anorexia one possibility is that a higher center is overriding the normal effectiveness of the hypothalamic area; another possibility is that some subtle disruption of the integrative mechanisms within the hypothalamus itself has resulted in a regulation error. In any case, obesity produced as a result of traumatic assault and destruction of part of the brain, while a useful preparation, must be considered a gross approximation of the physiological condition.

However, there are at least two ways in which VMH lesioned rats are like obese humans: obese humans, like VMH lesioned rats, do ingest more of a preferred food than normal-weight individuals, a factor that could be related to incorrect orosensory central integration; VMH lesioned rats (16), obese humans (47), and Zucker rats (48) show a disruption of their diurnal eating patterns. The meaning of this diurnal disruption is as yet unclear, but provides an interesting area for further investigation. The provocative finding that the obese Zucker rat does not show the behavior deficits previously attributed to VMH lesioned rats and extrapolated to humans, opens up another intriguing set of possibilities for developing new animal models of human obesity.

BEHAVIORAL CORRELATES OF ACTIVITY IN OBESE RATS AND HUMANS

While much attention has been focused on the caloric input component of the body weight regulation equation, many fewer attempts have been made to understand how caloric output is utilized by man or animals as a regulator. It is part of the conventional wisdom that obese humans are less active than their normal-weight counterparts. In fact, Bullen, Reed, and Mayer (49) were able to demonstrate that overweight adolescents placed in activity-producing situations managed to be less active than those of normal weight; for example, overweight girls during swim sessions at summer camp spent more time floating and less time actively swimming than normal-weight campers. Whether the decreased activity precedes or follows the onset of obesity, however, has yet to be clarified. It is certainly feasible to hypothesize that decreased activity and not increased caloric intake precedes the onset of obesity. Increases in body weight may further lessen the probability of sustained vigorous activity and lead to a propagation of the obese state both metabolically and morphologically. Since the pediatrician considers that increasing the activity of children and adolescents is a much less traumatic intervention than markedly reducing caloric intake, delineation of the factors that might lead to decreased activity in the early years of development is of particular concern.

Using the Zucker rat as a model for early-onset human obesity and examining the role of changes in activity in the genesis of obesity, Stern and Johnson (50) studied the spontaneous activity changes seen during the early postnatal development of lean and obese Zucker rats. They reported that Zucker obese and lean rat pups when given daily 3-hour access to activity wheels from 16 days of age until weaning run an equivalent amount of time in the wheels, but after weaning the lean animals continue to increase the amount of running time while the obese weanlings remain at their preweaning level of running or decline slightly. From day 16 to day 24 the obese pups weigh a small but significant amount more than the lean pups and eat more lab chow than the lean pups during the time when they are in the wheels and away from the nursing mother. These data seem to suggest that, at least in the Zucker rat, the onset of obesity precedes any change in the level of spontaneous activity. Wheel running in rats does vary with nutritional status, since rats deprived of food increase the amount they run (51) and the increase is proportional to the degree of deprivation (52). Furthermore, Bolles (53) has reported that rats run in wheels in anticipation of their daily feeding period when they are being fed on a two-meals-a-day schedule. Interpretation of wheel-running behaviors in rodents is difficult to extrapolate to humans because these particular behaviors in the laboratory rat could be associated with some vestigial pattern that might be adaptive in the wild (when dispersal of individuals in a situation of limited food supply would enhance the chance for survival) rather than with a mechanism involved in the regulation of body weight. Nonetheless, the spontaneous developmental differences seen between the obese and lean Zucker rats may provide a tool to detect changes in caloric output early in development, before gross obesity manifests itself. Potentially early manipulation of regulators associated with caloric output may be more permanent and less traumatic to the obese child than restriction of dietary intake or pharmacological intervention.

The multitude of behaviors associated with obesity substantiate the concept that obesity represents the pathological malfunction of a complex homeostatic mechanism regulating normal body weight. In a complex system there are many potential points for error and consequently many variants of the pathology. In the case of obesity, not only metabolism and morphology may be disrupted, but multiple behavioral correlates may emerge. Although the sheer complexity can occasionally overwhelm both experimenter and physician, the use of individualized behavioral analysis and behavioral modification techniques seems the most promising and rational approach to treatment at present. Perhaps with more elegant and extensive use of animal models and carefully controlled human studies an understanding of the variables associated with multifactoral regulation will be possible.

REFERENCES

1. J. Hirsch and J. Knittle, *Fed. Proc.* **29**: 1516 (1970).
2. P. R. Johnson, L. M. Zucker, S. A. F. Cruce, and J. Hirsch, *J. Lipid Res.* **12**: 706 (1971).
3. P. R. Johnson and J. Hirsch, *J. Lipid Res.* **13**: 2 (1972).
4. P. Bjorntorp, *Adv. Psychosom. Med.* **7**: 116 (1972).
5. S. Larsson, *Acta Physiol. Scand.* **52**: 171 (1961).
6. C. Baile and J. Mayer, *Science* **151**: 458 (1966).
7. H. D. Janowitz and M. I. Grossman, *Am. J. Physiol.* **158**: 184 (1949).
8. G. P. Smith and S. N. Epstein, *Am. J. Physiol.* **217**: 1083 (1969).
9. B. K. Anand and J. R. Brobeck, *Yale J. Biol. Med.* **24**: 123 (1951).
10. A. W. Hetherington and S. W. Ranson, *Anat. Rec.* **78**: 149 (1940).
11. J. Le Magnen, *Prog. Physiol. Psychol.* **4**: 22 (1970).
12. A. N. Epstein and P. Teitelbaum, *J. Comp. Physiol. Psychol.* **55**: 753 (1962).
13. G. L. Holman, *J. Comp. Physiol. Psychol.* **69**: 432 (1969).
14. J. Le Magnen, *Ann. N.Y. Acad. Sci.* **157**: 1126 (1969).
15. J. Le Magnen, *Adv. Psychosom. Med.* **7**: 73 (1972).
16. H. Kissileff, *Physiol. & Behav.* **5**: 163 (1972).
17. N. E. Miller, C. J. Bailey, and J. A. F. Stevenson, *Science* **112**: 256 (1950).

18. H. Graff and E. Stellar, *J. Comp. Physiol. Psychol.* **55**: 418 (1962).
19. H. L. Jacobs and K. N. Sharma, *Ann. N.Y. Acad. Sci.* **157**: 1084 (1969).
20. E. Becker, Presented at Eastern Psychological Assn., Boston, 1972.
21. P. Teitelbaum, *J. Comp. Physiol. Psychol.* **50**: 486 (1957).
22. M. R. C. Greenwood, P. R. Johnson, J. A. F. Cruce, and J. Hirsch, *Physiol. Behav.* **13**: 687 (1974).
23. J. A. F. Cruce, M. R. C. Greenwood, P. R. Johnson, and D. J. Quartermain, *J. Comp. Physiol. Psychol.* **87**: 295 (1974).
24. D. W. Pfaff, *Nature* **223**: 77 (1969).
25. S. Schachter, *Science* **161**: 171 (1968).
26. Nisbett, R. E. *Adv. Psychosom. Med.* **7**: 173 (1972).
27. R. E. Nisbett, *Science* **159**: 1254 (1968).
28. L. D. Ross, Doctoral Dissert. Columbia University (1970).
29. R. E. Nisbett, *J. Person. Soc. Psychol.* **10**: 107 (1968).
30. R. G. Campbell, S. Hashim, and T. B. Van Itallie, *N. Eng. J. Med.* **285**: 1402 (1971).
31. M. L. Glucksman and J. Hirsch, *Psychosom. Med.* **31**: 1 (1969).
32. M. L. Glucksman et al., *Psychosom. Med.* **30**: 359 (1968).
33. J. Grinker, M. L. Glucksman, J. Hirsch, and G. Viseltear, *Psychosom. Med.* **35**: 104 (1973).
34. J. Price and J. Grinker, *J. Comp. Physiol. Psychol.* **85**: 265 (1973).
35. J. Grinker, J. Hirsch, and D. Smith, *J. Person. Soc. Psychol.* **22**: 320 (1972).
36. O. W. Wooley, S. C. Wooley, and R. B. Dunham, *J. Comb. Physiol. Psychol.* **80**: 250 (1970).
37. B. W. Robinson and M. Mishkin, *Science* **136**: 260 (1962).
38. H. Graff and E. Stellar, *J. Comp. Physiol. Psychol.* **55**: 418 (1962).
39. R. Larkin, Doctoral Dissert., Rockefeller University (1973).
40. A. Sculfani and S. P. Grossman, *Physiol. & Behav.* **4**: 533 (1969).
41. J. Mendelson, *Science* **166**: 1431 (1969).
42. S. P. Grossman, *Adv. Psychosom. Med.* **7**: 49 (1972).
43. B. G. Hoebel and P. Teitelbaum, *J. Comp. Physiol. Psych.* **61**: 189 (1966).
44. T. L. Powley and R. E. Keesey, *J. Comp. Physiol. Psych.* **70**: 25 (1970).
45. E. Stellar, *Psychol. Rev.* **61**: 522 (1954).
46. J. Hirsch, *Adv. Psychosom. Med.* **7**: 229 (1969).
47. J. Grinker and J. Hirsch, in *Physiology and Emotion*, a Ciba Foundation Symposium, Amsterdam: Elsevier, 1972, p. 349.
48. E. Becker and H. Kissileff, *Physiol. Behav.* (In press).
49. B. A. Bullen, R. B. Reed, and J. Mayer, *Am. J. Clin. Nutr.* **14**: 211 (1964).
50. J. S. Stern and P. R. Johnson, *Fed. Proc.* **33**: 677 (1974).
51. J. S. Hall, K. Smith, S. B. Schnitzer and P. F. Hanford, *J. Comp. Physiol. Psychol.* **46**: 429 (1953).
52. M. J. Moskowitz, *Comp. Physiol. Psychol.* **52**: 621 (1959).
53. R. C. Bolles and S. A. Moot, *J. Comp. Physiol. Psychol.* **83**: 510 (1973).

Index

Abdominal Colic, 95
Acidosis, respiratory, 160
Acquired hypercholesterolemia, 104
Acromegalic patients, 158
Activities, 71
Activity, 77, 143, 145
  behavior associated with, 163
  decreased, 71, 173
  physical, 6, 129, 145, 148
  spontaneous, 173
Adipocyte(s), 1, 2, 11, 15, 16, 20
  division, 11
  DNA in, 19
  mature, 19
  pool, 19
  insulin sensitivity, 138
Adipose cells, 139
  enlargment, 136
Adipose cell number, 1, 2, 11, 15-17,
    19, 135, 136, 138
Adipose cell size, 1, 2, 15, 136, 138
Adipose cellularity, 16, 18, 20
Adipose depot(s), 4, 18, 172
  morphology, 168
  reduction, 172
  saturated fat in, 4
Adipose tissue, 1, 86
  critical periods in development, 3,
    84, 137
  epinephrine, 138
  fetal, 4
  growth hormone, 138
  hyperplasia, 81
  insulin, 138
  mobilization, 47
  modification, 50

morphology, 15
  regulatory dysfunction, 168
  sex-related difference, 82
Adiposity, degree of, 61
Adolescence, 7, 32, 82
  body mass, 82
Adolescent, obese, 6
Adolescent period, adipose tissue
    development, 84, 137
Adoption, 76
Adult obesity, 40
Adult-onset obesity, 169
Adenyl cyclase, 139
Affection, 142
African, 40
Age, 61
Age of onset of obesity, 168
Albumin, 50
American blacks, 33, 35, 37
American whites, 32, 37
Amphetamines, 155
Anabolic period, 7, 86
Aneurism, aortic, 114
Angina, 97, 157
  pectoris, 115
Animal fats, 94
Animal models of obesity, 172
Anorexia, 172
Anti-insulin properties, 75
Anxiety, 147
Aorta, human, 113
Aortic, aneurism, 114
Aortic ejection murmur, 97
Appendectomies, 84
Appetite, child's, 129
  increase, 155